TALKING POINTS
IN DERMATOLOGY – II

Presented to

----

with the compliments of

----

your Upjohn Representative

As a service to medical education **Upjohn**

Other titles in the *New Clinical Applications* Series:

Dermatology (Series Editor Dr J. L. Verbov)
Dermatological Surgery
Superficial Fungal Infections
Talking Points in Dermatology – I
Treatment in Dermatology
Current Concepts in Contact Dermatitis

Cardiology (Series Editor Dr D. Longmore)
Cardiology Screening

Rheumatology (Series Editors Dr J. J. Calabro and Dr W. Carson Dick)
Ankylosing Spondylitis
Infections and Arthritis

Nephrology (Series Editor Dr G. R. D. Catto)
Continuous Ambulatory Peritoneal Dialysis
Management of Renal Hypertension
Chronic Renal Failure
Calculus Disease
Pregnancy and Renal Disorders
Multisystem Diseases
Glomerulonephritis I
Glomerulonephritis II

NEW
CLINICAL
APPLICATIONS
DERMATOLOGY

TALKING POINTS IN DERMATOLOGY – II

Editor

JULIAN L. VERBOV
JP, MD, FRCP, FIBiol

Consultant Dermatologist
Royal Liverpool Hospital,
Liverpool, UK

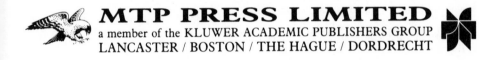

MTP PRESS LIMITED
a member of the KLUWER ACADEMIC PUBLISHERS GROUP
LANCASTER / BOSTON / THE HAGUE / DORDRECHT

Published in the UK and Europe by
MTP Press Limited
Falcon House
Lancaster, England

British Library Cataloguing in Publication Data

Talking points in dermatology.—(New
 clinical applications. Dermatology; v. 6).
 2
 1. Dermatology
 I. Verbov, Julian   II. Series
 616.5   RL71

 ISBN 0–85200–689–6
 ISBN 0–85200–823–6 series

Published in the USA by
MTP Press
A division of Kluwer Boston Inc
190 Old Derby Street
Hingham, MA 02043, USA

Library of Congress Cataloging-in-Publication Data

Talking points in dermatology—II.

 (New clinical applications. Dermatology)
 Includes bibliographies and index.
 1. Dermatology.   2. AIDS (Disease).   3. Opportunistic
infections.   4. Photodermatitis.   5. Pruritus.
6. Trace elements in the body.   7. Skin—Diseases—
Psychosomatic aspects.   I. Verbov, Julian.   II. Title:
Talking points in dermatology—2.   III. Series.
[DNLM: 1. Skin Diseases.   WR 140 T146]
RL87.T35   1987   616.5   87–22624
ISBN 0–85200–689–6

Typeset and printed by Butler & Tanner Ltd,
Frome and London

CONTENTS

LIST OF AUTHORS

Dr J. A. Cotterill, MD, FRCP
Consultant Dermatologist
The General Infirmary at Leeds
Leeds
LS1 3EX

Dr R. M. Graham, MB, MRCP
Senior Registrar
Department of Dermatology
Royal Liverpool Hospital
Prescot Street
Liverpool
L7 8XP

Dr J. L. M. Hawk, MRCP,
FRACP
Consultant Dermatologist
Photobiology Unit
11th Floor, North Wing
St Thomas' Hospital
London
SE1 7EH

Dr M. M. Molokhia, MD
Consultant Dermatologist
Halton General Hospital
Runcorn
Cheshire
WA7 2DA

Dr M. F. Muhlemann, BSc,
MRCP
Consultant Dermatologist
Dept. of Dermatology
The General Hospital
St. Helier
Jersey
Channel Islands

SERIES EDITOR'S FOREWORD

This is Volume 6 of the popular series updating selected topics in dermatology.

As usual the authors have a particular interest in their subject. Dr Muhlemann opens with an excellent review on the skin in HIV infection. Dr Hawk then presents an authoritative chapter on light eruptions. A comprehensive and informative chapter by Dr Graham on itching follows. Dr Molokhia brings his particular expertise to trace elements in dermatology and finally Dr Cotterill provides a sparkling, succinct contribution on the skin and the psyche.

JULIAN VERBOV

ABOUT THE EDITOR

Dr Julian Verbov is Consultant Dermatologist to Liverpool Health Authority and Clinical Lecturer in Dermatology at the University of Liverpool.

He is a member of the British Association of Dermatologists representing the British Society for Paediatric Dermatology on its Executive Committee. He is a Council Member of the Dermatology Section of the Royal Society of Medicine, and a Committee Member of the North of England Dermatological Society.

He is a Fellow of the Zoological Society of London and a Member of the Society of Authors. He is a popular speaker and author of more than 190 publications. His special interests include paediatric dermatology, inherited disorders, dermatoglyphics, pruritus ani, therapeutics, and medical humour. He organizes the British Postgraduate Course in Paediatric Dermatology and is a Member of the Editorial Boards of both *Clinical and Experimental Dermatology* and *Pediatric Dermatology*.

1

THE SKIN IN HIV INFECTION

M. F. MUHLEMANN

THE ACQUIRED IMMUNODEFICIENCY SYNDROME

The acquired immunodeficiency syndrome (AIDS) has now reached epidemic proportions and is worldwide. Within the next few years there will be few physicians in Britain who will not have had first hand experience of dealing with or diagnosing patients with AIDS. The number of affected patients in the United Kingdom is, at the time of writing, still fortunately small but the potential number of AIDS victims based on the prevalence of Human Immunodeficiency Virus (HIV) antibody amongst at risk individuals is alarming. Although the exact number of cases cannot be predicted from the antibody prevalence, large numbers appear to be inevitable.

AIDS is caused by HIV, a retrovirus in which RNA transcription proceeds in a reverse direction before incorporation of the viral genome into the host genome. This action requires a reverse transcriptase enzyme. The virus is specifically lymphotropic for the thymus dependant (T) helper lymphocytes and as a result patients with HIV infection may exhibit defects in cell-mediated immunity. Patients with AIDS have a reduction in absolute numbers of T helper lymphocytes with a decrease in the T helper/suppressor ratio (T_H/T_S), hyper-gammaglobulinaemia and an impaired response to common recall antigens.

AIDS is defined as the occurrence of a reliably diagnosed disease that is at least moderately indicative of underlying cellular immune deficiency in a patient with no known cause other than HIV infection

TABLE 1.1 Diseases moderately predictive for underlying defect in cell mediated immunity

---

Viral
　　Cytomegalovirus – lung, gut or CNS.
　　Herpes simplex – severe mucocutaneous for longer than 1 month, lung, gut or disseminated.
　　Progressive multifocal leukoencephalopathy

Protozoal
　　Pneumocystis carinii pneumonia
　　Toxoplasmosis – pneumonia, CNS
　　Cryptosporidiosis and Isosporiasis – prolonged diarrhoea
　　Strongyloidosis – lung, CNS or disseminated

Fungal
　　Candidiasis – lung or oesophageal
　　Cryptococcosis – lung, CNS or disseminated
　　Histoplasmosis – disseminated
　　Aspergillosis – lung or disseminated

Bacterial
　　Atypical mycobacteria other than *M. tuberculosis*

Neoplastic
　　Cerebral lymphoma
　　Kaposi's sarcoma
　　Non-Hodgkins lymphoma

Miscellaneous
　　Chronic interstitial pneumonitis in children

---

for such, nor any other cause of reduced resistance reported to be associated with that disease[1]. Diseases indicative of an underlying cellular immune deficiency are listed in Table 1.1. Patients are excluded from this diagnosis if they are seronegative for antibody to HIV, have no other positive tests for other HIV infections and do not have a low ratio of T helper to T suppressor lymphocytes. The proportion of those infected with HIV who ultimately progress to AIDS is unknown but the percentage is gradually increasing as more cases are recorded with longer incubation times. This may vary from eight months to eight years. The outcome of HIV infection will depend on the host's ability to mount an immune response and it is this response that results in the spectrum of disease caused by infection with HIV. Many patients

2

will remain asymptomatic, some will develop persistent generalized lymphadenopathy (PGL), others will develop AIDS-related complex (ARC) and others AIDS.

PGL is defined as lymphadenopathy for longer than three months at two or more extrainguinal sites in the absence of any other illness known to cause lymphadenopathy. The definition of ARC is the presence of any two of the following clinical findings: fatigue, night sweats, lymphadenopathy longer than three months, weight loss, fever longer than three months or diarrhoea combined with two of the following laboratory findings: decreased T helper cell count, increased serum globulins and anergy. Progression from PGL to ARC and ultimately to AIDS may be documented in the same patient and is associated with a decline in immune function but this is by no means inevitable.

SKIN DISEASE WITH HIV INFECTION

The dermatological hallmark of AIDS is Kaposi's sarcoma (KS) and it was this previously uncommon tumour occurring in young fit homosexual men that alerted physicians to the AIDS epidemic[2]. Chronic ulcerative perianal herpes simplex and oral and oesophageal candidiasis are other dermatological manifestations which have become reliably predictive for the development of AIDS. Other infective and non-infective dermatoses are regularly found with PGL, ARC and AIDS and whilst they are not diagnostic of AIDS they are regarded by many to be strongly predictive of an underlying defect of cellular immunity and should prompt further immunological investigation. These will be discussed individually in this chapter along with a review of the current literature concerning other dermatoses that have been reported in association with HIV infection.

Acute HIV infection

The earliest skin manifestation of HIV infection is a roseola-like rash associated with an acute infectious mononucleosis-like illness. During a prospective immuno-epidemiological study of homosexual men,

3

acute HIV seroconversion was documented in 11 patients in whom there was a sudden onset of an illness lasting between 3 to 14 days accompanied by a macular erythematous eruption on the face, trunk and limbs and which involved the palms and soles[3]. Other symptoms included fever, malaise, anorexia, lethargy, headache, sore throat, myalgia, arthralgia and diarrhoea. Generalized lymphadenopathy was also found. Laboratory tests showed an inverted T_H/T_S ratio, lymphopenia, thrombocytopenia and HIV seroconversion.

Kaposi's sarcoma

Until the emergence of AIDS, Kaposi's sarcoma (KS) was only rarely encountered in the western world and affected elderly Mediterranean patients often of Jewish stock and occasionally immunosuppressed patients. In equatorial Africa, in particular Uganda, Zambia and Zaire, classical KS is endemic and found in a similar geographical distribution as Burkitt's lymphoma. Classical KS is a slow-growing indolent vascular tumour that most commonly arises on the lower limbs and may take many years before it metastasizes. Four clinical subtypes are recognized in classical KS. Nodular tumours account for 85% of lesions and are associated with the most favourable prognosis. Ulcerative, infiltrative and generalized forms are less common and more aggressive.

Serology of Kaposi's sarcoma

Patients with classical KS, KS associated with other forms of immunosuppression and endemic African KS are seronegative for HIV. Aggressive forms of African KS associated with opportunistic infections and immunodeficiency are HIV positive and are clinically similar to KS in western AIDS patients. Generally, these aggressive forms account for about 10% of African cases and are most often found in the areas where endemic HIV infection overlaps with the regions

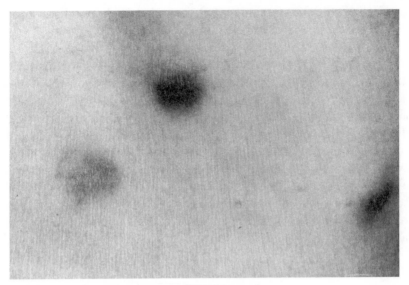

FIGURE 1.1   Kaposi's sarcomata on the trunk

where non-HIV KS is endemic such as Zambia and Uganda.

In contrast to classical KS, AIDS associated KS behaves in a more aggressive manner. Although lesions may begin on the lower limbs, the more usual presentation is of a widespread eruption of discrete purple-red nodules on the trunk, upper limbs and face (Figure 1.1). Lesions are often linear and follow the skin lines. They may coalesce in later stages to form larger plaques. Sites most commonly affected on the head and neck are the nose, eyelids and oropharynx (Figures 1.2, 1.3) and examination of the latter is mandatory in any patient with skin disease and positive HIV serology. Diagnosis of early lesions can be very difficult. Lesions may begin as a faint macular vascular blush and the diagnosis will only become apparent as lesions gradually darken, thicken and pigment as haemosiderin is deposited in dermal macrophages. KS may mimic amelanotic melanoma, histiocytoma and pyogenic granuloma. It is probable that KS is derived from lymphatic endothelium. Immunocytochemical studies using the monoclonal antibodies EN4, a marker for endothelium of vascular and lymphatic origin, and PALE, a marker for vascular endothelium,

5

have indicated that lymphangiomatous and probably nodular KS are derived from lymphatic endothelium[4].

Patients who develop KS as the only manifestation of AIDS tend to have a better prognosis than those who present with opportunistic infection. KS also occurs more frequently in male homosexuals than in any other risk group. Although KS is a radiosensitive tumour and occasionally may show spontaneous regression, the usual outcome is of spread to the lymph nodes and internal organs. The gastrointestinal tract is commonly affected. Lymphoedema is a frequent accompaniment when regional lymph nodes are involved. Patients with AIDS usually die from overwhelming opportunistic infection rather than from metastatic KS but occasionally they succumb from gastrointestinal haemorrhage from a lesion of KS or to pulmonary infiltration by KS.

Treatment

Cosmetically disfiguring solitary lesions may be surgically excised or treated by paliative local radiotherapy. If lesions are more numerous they may respond to electron beam therapy or intralesional chemotherapy with vinblastine. Systemic chemotherapy is best avoided as it will worsen immunosuppression and adversely affect the prognosis.

SKIN INFECTION IN HIV DISEASE

Virus infection

The underlying susceptibility to infection in AIDS is undoubtedly due to the depletion of T helper lymphocytes but, in addition, natural killer cell function and blastogenic responsiveness to mitogens and antigens are impaired. Decreased numbers of HLA-DR positive Langerhans cells are also found in the skin. Virus infection in AIDS is commonplace, particularly with the double stranded DNA viruses. Skin and mucosal infection has been reported with the herpetoviridae, papovaviridae and poxviridae.

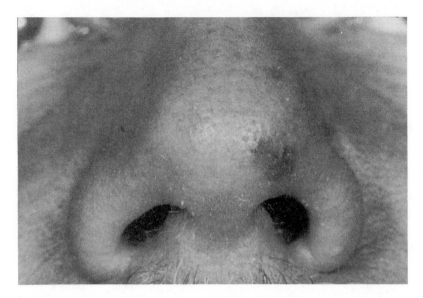

FIGURE 1.2   Kaposi's sarcoma on the tip of the nose

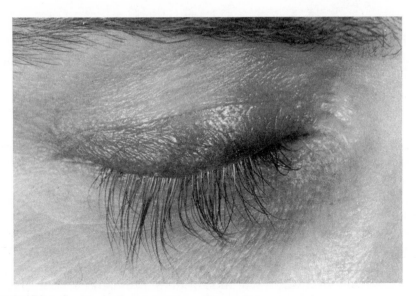

FIGURE 1.3   Kaposi's sarcoma on the eyelid

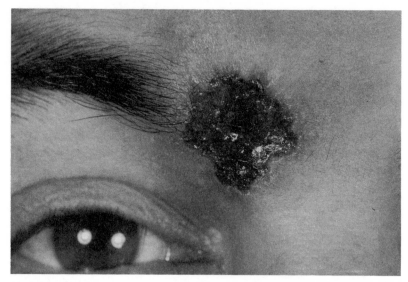

FIGURE 1.4   Chronic herpes simplex on the face in a patient with ARC

Herpes simplex

Attacks of herpes simplex virus type I (HSVI) are common in patients who are immunosuppressed but also occur in normal subjects who have intercurrent infection, in the elderly and with sun exposure and PUVA therapy as a consequence of depressed immune function. It is therefore not surprising that HSVI and HSVII infections are more common in patients with PGL, ARC and AIDS (Figure 1.4). In 1981, Siegal[5] reported severe, chronic perianal HSV infection in male homosexuals with acquired immunodeficiency. This form of HSV infection is now regarded as pathognomonic for infection with HIV and occurs most often in this risk group.

HSVII and HSVI cause genital herpes. The increased number of cases of genital herpes caused by HSVI reflects the increase in oro-genital sexual behaviour. Both virus types give rise to identical symp-toms and signs. Sites affected are the glans penis, shaft of penis, pubic region, perianal skin, anus and rectum. Early symptoms are of malaise, anorexia and fever with a sensation of burning or paraesthesiae in the affected area. This is followed by multiple, small vesicular and pustular

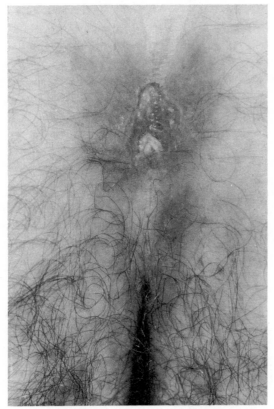

FIGURE 1.5   Chronic perianal ulcerative herpes simplex

lesions which develop on an erythematous base and progress to ulceration. Lesions are exquisitely tender and when they affect the urethra or anal margin are accompanied by dysuria and acute anorectal pain. Tender, local lymphadenopathy is usual and secondary bacterial infection is common. Involvement of the sacral nerves may give rise to urinary retention.

Recurrent genital HSV infections are generally less severe except for the chronic recurrent perianal form seen in homosexuals with HIV infection (Figure 1.5). Diagnosis should be confirmed wherever possible by virus culture or electron microscopy and infections treated with acyclovir, an antiviral agent specific for herpes infection. Treat-

9

ment with acyclovir will reduce viral shedding times and decrease morbidity but unfortunately does not reduce time to recurrence. Attention should be paid to secondary bacterial infection and when present it should be treated with systemic antibacterials and topical antiseptics.

Herpes Zoster

There is now ample evidence that varicella zoster virus also occurs more commonly in HIV infection. A study of patients with ophthalmic herpes zoster showed that it occurred more often in at-risk groups for AIDS, and was associated with lymphopenia and inversion of T_H/T_S, than in non-risk patients who had normal T cell ratios[6]. Freidman-Klein *et al*[7] in a retrospective study of 300 patients with AIDS documented that 8% had had prior zoster. In a prospective study of 48 consecutive patients with thoracic zoster, 85% had risk factors for AIDS and 72% were HIV positive. The HIV positive group had depressed T cell ratios and impaired lymphocyte mitogen responses. Seven patients subsequently developed AIDS and one patient seroconverted. The authors considered that herpes zoster was a sign of depressed cellular immunity and may herald the onset of ARC or AIDS. Symptoms and signs are no different than in the non-immunosuppressed, although more than one dermatome may be affected simultaneously and recurrences may occur.

Human papilloma virus

The human papilloma virus (HPV) is ubiquitous and affects all age groups. Immunosuppressed renal transplant recipients have a high incidence of genital and non-genital viral warts, the prevalence of which increases with the length of time of immunosuppression[8]. Genital and non-genital warts are also common in homosexual at-risk

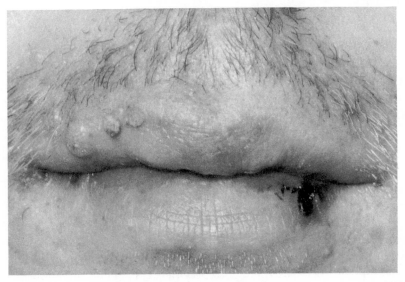

FIGURE 1.6   HPV labial warts and angular cheilitis in patient with AIDS

patients (Figure 1.6). Although it is the author's impression that genital warts are no more common in male homosexuals with HIV infection, no prevalence studies are available to confirm or refute this impression. However, genital warts in patients with HIV may become extensive, exophytic and more resistant to therapy.

Molluscum contagiosum

This double-stranded DNA-containing poxvirus is reported to occur with increased frequency in patients receiving chemotherapy and steroids, and with sarcoidosis and eczema, conditions that are associated with depressed cellular immune function. Now there have been several reports of severe, widespread and chronic molluscum contagiosum infections in patients with AIDS. Infections particularly affect the head and neck[9]. Restriction enzyme analysis of viral DNA reveals that there are two types of molluscum virus. These subtypes do not show a predilection for one particular clinical site unlike the HSV (unpublished) but whether this is true for patients with AIDS is uncertain.

11

Oral 'hairy' leukoplakia

Hairy leukoplakia is not an uncommon finding in patients with HIV disease and when seen in patients with ARC carries a poor prognosis. Leukoplakia characteristically affects the lateral borders of the tongue and has a corrugated and hairy appearance. It is rarely symptomatic. Histopathological changes show koilocytosis and a tufted acanthosis. Papillomavirus core antigen, herpes virus-like particles and Epstein-Barr virus have all been found in association with hairy leukoplakia in male homosexuals with HIV associated immunodeficiency[10].

Bacterial infection

Streptococcal and staphylococcal skin infection are seen more often in patients with PGL, ARC and AIDS. Erysipelas and cellulitis are usually due to *Streptococcus pyogenes,* a group A haemolytic strep-tococcus but in immunosuppressed patients groups B, C and G may be implicated. The diagnostic morphological clues may be absent or difficult to recognize in these patients so that the typical erythema may be absent, the eruption may be ill-defined or the oedema develop long before the pyrexia. Infection with streptococcal groups B, C and G may account for some of these diagnostic difficulties[11]. Staphylococcal impetigo is also a frequent finding. The author has seen several cases of curiously localized chronic impetigo that affected the whole of the beard area in patients with PGL and ARC[12]. Treatment with systemic antibiotics is usually successful but infections tend to recur, especially if the patient is a carrier of *Staphylococcus aureus.*

Fungal infection

Candidiasis

Oral and oesophageal candidiasis is an established finding in patients with HIV infection. Patients with ARC frequently have oral lesions but when it involves the oesophagus the patient is regarded as having AIDS. Lesions may occur as thick white plaques or as a scant white exudate on an angry inflamed buccal mucosa and posterior pharynx

12

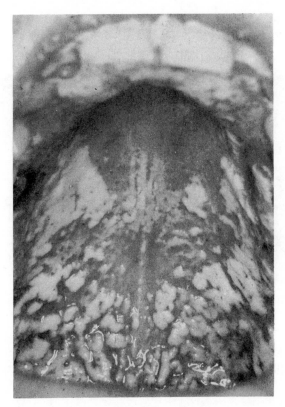

FIGURE 1.7   Oral candidiasis in AIDS

(Figure 1.7). Dysphagia is a common symptom when there are oeso-phageal lesions. Klein showed that oral candidiasis was a frequent finding in patients at risk for AIDS and when found in the presence of a reversed T_H/T_S ratio was strongly predictive for AIDS[13]. By way of a contrast, patients with PGL and a reversed T_H/T_S ratio but without candida did not progress to AIDS. *Candida albicans* is usually the causative species but occasionally others may be isolated. Candida may also be cultured from hairy leukoplakia, angular cheilitis and nail dystrophy. Oral candidiasis can be partially controlled by nystatin suspension or amphotericin lozenges but quickly relapses when treat-

13

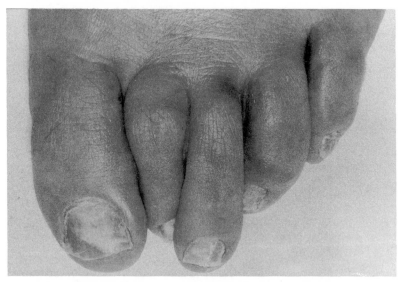

FIGURE 1.8   *T. rubrum* infection of toenails. Note KS in toe web spaces

ment is stopped. Oesophageal candidiasis is very resistant to therapy and may require long term treatment with oral ketoconazole.

Dermatophyte infection

Extensive and florid dermatophyte infections are a striking feature in patients with HIV infection and may also be regarded as a poor prognostic indicator[12]. Trichophyton, Epidermophyton and Microsporon species have been recovered from the skin, hair and nails of AIDS patients. It is not uncommon for patients to have coexisting infections of the nails (Figure 1.8), feet, groins and trunk. Marked erythema, scaling and pustulation is usually present. Griseofulvin and ketoconazole may not be effective and relapse is frequent.

Histoplasmosis

Disseminated histoplasmosis caused by the yeast *Histoplasma capsulatum* is now pathognomonic for AIDS in high-risk patients who have HIV antibodies[14]. Oral or skin manifestations occur in 6% of patients with disseminated histoplasmosis and may present as papules, nodules, plaques, pustules, abscesses or ulcers. Dermatitis, oral nodules with ulceration, erythroderma and panniculitis have also occurred with disseminated histoplasmosis. Diagnosis may be confirmed by finding the yeast in skin biopsies but it may be cultured from almost any tissue. The yeast is round or oval with budding bodies and may be seen surrounded by a clear halo within macrophages. Histoplasma stains with PAS, methenamine silver or Giemsa. The characteristic granulomatous histology is often absent in patients with depressed cellular immunity but abundant yeast forms may be seen in the dermis. Recurrence or persistence is usual in AIDS and the prognosis is poor. The treatment of choice is either systemic amphotericin B or ketoconazole.

Other fungus infections

Cutaneous *Cryptococcus neoformans* infection that resembled molluscum contagiosum was present in one patient with AIDS[15] and in another patient, cutaneous and systemic cryptococcosis was found in association with torulopsis and epidermodysplasia veruciformis[16].

Seborrhoeic dermatitis, pityrosporon folliculitis and folliculitis

These disorders are considered together as there is now increasing evidence to implicate the yeast *Pityrosporon ovale* in their pathogenesis. In 1984, Eisenstat and Wormser[17] reported an increased incidence of seborrhoeic dermatitis in patients with AIDS. I have found a statistically significant increase in seborrhoeic dermatitis in male homosexuals with PGL when compared to an HIV-negative control group of male homosexuals. This finding was not seen in asymptomatic HIV-positive patients when compared with negative controls[12]. A

15

striking feature of the seborrhoeic dermatitis is the florid nature of the eruption, which occurs in a butterfly distribution on the cheeks (Figure 1.9). This may have distinct histological features, with keratinocyte necrosis and a dermal infiltrate composed of plasma cells and neutrophils with leukocytoclasia[18]. Lesions may be widespread and are sometimes associated with an intensely itchy follicular erythematous papular and pustular eruption affecting the face, back and upper chest (Figure 1.10). Bacteriological culture of the follicular pustules are consistently negative but the histology may show a severe mixed peri-follicular and follicular inflammatory infiltrate of lymphocytes, neutrophils, eosinophils and plasma cells often with abundant *P. ovale* yeasts within the follicle. Pityrosporon folliculitis, although frequently found in association with seborrhoeic dermatitis, may occur independently.

There are patients who have a generalized follicular eruption who do not have pityrosporon folliculitis. In this group, the folliculitis usually begins on the face and spreads to the upper chest, back, arms, axillae, thighs and buttocks (Figures 1.11, 1.12). The follicular papules develop on a background of low-grade erythema and with the development of severe pruritus there is xerosis, eczematization and secondary infection. This type of folliculitis has been seen by the author in patients at high risk for AIDS and with PGL, all of whom developed AIDS, and is regarded as a poor prognostic sign[12]. A recurrence of teenage acne or an exacerbation of acne has been noted in patients with PGL and ARC. In a recent report of folliculitis in a patient with ARC, the histological appearances were those of a necrotizing folliculitis with a neutrophil infiltrate, necrosis of the follicular wall and a fibrinoid necrosis of accompanying small vessels[19].

Pityrosporon yeasts were found by McGinley *et al* to be more abundant in the scalp flora of patients with pityriasis capitis and seborrhoeic dermatitis than in normals[20]. Seborrhoeic dermatitis responds to treatment with topical and oral ketoconazole and provides a strong causal relationship[21]. It is possible that patients with acquired immunodeficiency are unable to prevent the overgrowth of pityrosporon yeasts and as a result they develop a folliculitis and seborrhoeic dermatitis. This might explain why no difference was found in the prevalence of seborrhoeic dermatitis in asymptomatic HIV-positive patients when compared with HIV-negative controls. Arguments

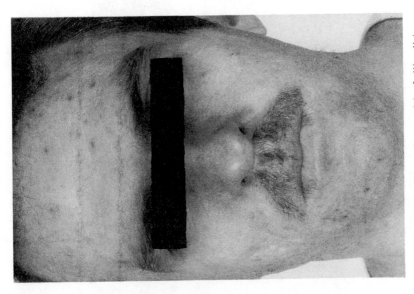

FIGURE 1.10 Chronic pruritic folliculitis on forehead in patient with ARC

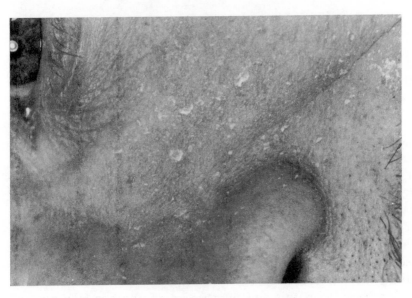

FIGURE 1.9 Seborrhoeic dermatitis in AIDS

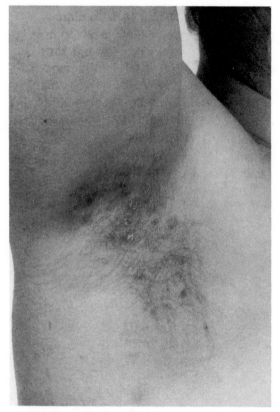

FIGURE 1.11   Axillary folliculitis in AIDS

against this hypothesis are that patients with seborrhoeic dermatitis in remission still have large numbers of *P. ovale* and that after clearance of the skin with selenium sulphide and topical amphotericin B there may be a prompt relapse of seborrhoeic dermatitis. It is possible that the yeast plays a secondary aggravating role by activating complement and thereby the inflammatory response. Of interest is that patients with **AIDS** given ketoconazole for oesophageal candidiasis or for folliculitis do not always improve and may develop seborrhoeic dermatitis whilst on treatment.

Seborrhoeic dermatitis and pityrosporon folliculitis may respond to topical imidazoles combined with topical steroids. In the author's

18

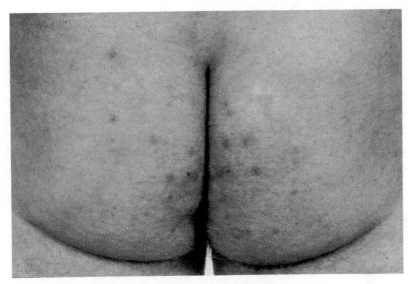

FIGURE 1.12   Folliculitis of the buttocks in AIDS

experience oral ketoconazole is seldom suppressive and should be used in conjunction with topical therapy. Eczema will respond to topical steroids but systemic antibiotics, emollients and antipruritics are usually needed.

ORAL CAVITY DISEASE

Examination of the mouth in patients who are known to be at risk or who are HIV antibody positive is important as many diagnostic clues may be uncovered. KS frequently affects the palate and posterior pharynx, leukoplakia may be seen on the tongue and there may be candidiasis and intraoral warts. Dental caries and dental abscesses are usual in AIDS patients. Non-specific findings include a coated tongue, aphthous ulceration and angular cheilitis.

19

VASCULITIS

Immune complex and allergic vasculitis have been documented in patients with AIDS[12,22]. One patient presented with Henoch–Schonlein purpura, was noted to have widespread folliculitis and fungal infection and subsequently developed AIDS. A second patient developed vasculitis and had a positive tissue indirect immunofluorescence of dermal blood vessels when using serum with a high titre of HIV antibody. This finding suggested that the virus was acting as the source of the antigen in the immune complex vasculitis.

PSORIASIS

Exacerbation of long-standing psoriasis has been seen in some patients with AIDS[23]. Progression to erythroderma occurred in 2 patients with psoriasis and in one patient erythrodermic psoriasis began at the time of the diagnosis of AIDS. This is an interesting observation that lends support to the theory that psoriasis may be an immunologically mediated disease. Reiter's syndrome may occur in HIV disease with typical hyperkeratotic rupioid lesions on the lower limbs, palms and soles and with mucosal lesions.

DRUG ERUPTIONS

Allergic hypersensitivity to co-trimoxazole occurs in up to 60% of patients who are being treated with this drug for pneumocystis carinii pneumonia. The patient will develop a fever, malaise and a maculopapular rash which becomes exfoliative. It is not known why patients with AIDS should develop this increased drug hypersensitivity.

MISCELLANEOUS FINDINGS IN HIV DISEASE

AIDS is a chronic, debilitating disease punctuated by bouts of opportunistic infections. Weight loss is gradual at first but in the late stages most patients are markedly cachectic and the skin becomes xerotic and sometimes ichthyotic. Patchy alopecia and premature greying are common as is the appearance of premature ageing. Pressure sores and chronic pyoderma may be troublesome nursing problems[24].

The yellow nail syndrome has developed in AIDS patients with chronic pulmonary tuberculosis, pleural effusions and sinusitis[25]. Pyoderma gangrenosum has occurred in a patient with asymptomatic HIV infection[26] and three patients developed the uncommon syndrome of eosinophilic pustular folliculitis[27]. This unusual condition is characterized by follicular papules and pustules on the face, trunk and proximal limbs which become confluent polycyclic indurated plaques. Lastly, a novel condition known as hyperalgesic pseudo-thrombophlebitis has been seen HIV positive male homosexuals who had a painful swelling of the leg with a tender overlying erythema that mimicked thrombophlebitis[28].

In summary, patients with HIV infection may develop an infectious mononucleosis-like illness at the time of seroconversion but remain asymptomatic until there is a decline in cell-mediated immunity and the development of PGL, ARC or AIDS. The cutaneous hallmark of AIDS is KS but viral, bacterial and fungal infections are common and may be reasonably predictive for AIDS when a reversal of the T_H/T_S is found. It is the recurrent, persistent and florid nature of these relatively innocuous disorders that should alert the physician to investigate the possibility of an underlying acquired immunodeficiency disorder.

References

1. Centres for Disease Control (1982a) Update on acquired immune deficiency syndrome (AIDS). *MMWR.*, **31**, 507–14
2. Friedman-Klein, A. E., Lanbenstein, L. J., Rubenstein, P. *et al.* (1982). Disseminated Kaposi's sarcoma in homosexual men. *Ann Intern Med.*, **96**, 693–9
3. Cooper, D. A., Gold, J., Maclean, P. *et al.* (1985). Acute AIDS retrovirus infection. *Lancet,* **1**, 537–40
4. Russell-Jones, R., Spaull, J., Spry, C. & Wilson-Jones, E. (1986). Histiogenesis of Kaposi's sarcoma in patients with and without immune deficiency syndrome (AIDS). *J. Clin. Pathol.*, **39**, 742–9
5. Siegal, F. P., Lopez, C., Hammer, G. S. *et al.* (1981) Severe acquired immunodeficiency in male homosexuals, manifested by chronic perianal ulcerative herpes simplex lesions. *N. Engl. J. Med.*, **305**, 1439–44
6. Sandor, E., Croxon, T. S., Millman, A. & Mildvan, D. (1984). Herpes zoster

ophthalmicus in patients at risk for AIDS. *N. Engl. J. Med.,* **310,** 1118

7. Friedman-Klein, A. E., Lafleur, P. L., Gendler, E. *et al.* (1986). Herpes zoster: A possible early clinical sign for the development of acquired immunodeficiency syndrome in high risk individuals. *J. Am. Acad. Dermatol.,* **14,** 1023–8

8. Rudlinger, R., Smith, I. W., Bunney, M. H. & Hunter, J. A. A. (1986). Human papillomavirus infections in a group of renal transplant recipients. *Br. J. Dermatol.,* **115,** 681–92

9. Redfield, R. R., James, W. D., Wright, D. C. *et al.* (1985) Severe molluscum contagiosum in a patient with human T cell lymphotrophic (HTLV III) disease. *J. Am. Acad. Dermatol.,* **13,** 821–4

10. Greenspan, D., Greenspan, J., Conant, M., Peterson, V., Silverman, S. Jr. & DeSouza, Y. (1984). Oral 'hairy' leukoplakia in male homosexuals. Evidence of association with both papillomavirus and herpes group virus. *Lancet,* **2,** 831–4

11. Cupps, T. R., Cotton, D. J., Schooley, R. T. & Fauei, A. S. (1981). Facial erysipelas in the immunocompromised host. *Arch. Dermatol.,* **117,** 47–9

12. Muhlemann, M. F., Anderson, M. G., Paradinas, F. J. *et al.* (1986). Early warning skin signs in patients with AIDS and persistent generalized lymphadenopathy. *Br. J. Dermatol.,* **114,** 419–24

13. Klein, R. S., Harris, C. A., Small, C. B., Moll, B., Lesser, M. & Friedland, G. H. (1984). Oral candidiasis in high risk patients as the initial manifestation of the acquired immunodeficiency syndrome. *N. Eng. J. Med.,* **311,** 354–8

14. Hazelhurst, J. A. & Vismer, H. F. (1985) Histoplasmosis presenting with unusual skin lesions in acquired immunodeficiency syndrome (AIDS). *Br. J. Dermatol.,* **113,** 345–8

15. Rico, M. J. & Penneys, N. S. (1985). Cutaneous cryptococcosis resembling molluscum contagiosum in a patient with AIDS. *Arch. Dermatol.,* **121,** 901–2

16. Grimm I (1984). Cutaneous and pulmonary cryptococcosis and torulopsidosis and epidermodysplasia verruciformis in AIDS. *Hautarzt,* **35,** 653–5

17. Eisenstat, B. A. & Wormser, G. P. (1984). Seborrhoeic dermatitis and butterfly rash in AIDS. *N. Engl. J. Med.,* **311,** 189

18. Soeprono, F. F., Schinella, R. A., Cockerell, C. J. and Comite, S. L. (1986). Seborrhoeic-like dermatitis of acquired immunodeficiency syndrome. *J. Am. Acad. Dermatol.,* **14,** 242–4

19. Barlow, R. J. and Schulz, E. J. (1987). Necrotizing folliculitis in AIDS-related complex. *Br. J. Dermatol.,* **116,** 581–4

20. McGinley, K. J., Leyden, J. J., Marples, R. R. & Kligman, A. M. (1975). Quantitative microbiology of the scalp in non-dandruff, dandruff and seborrhoeic dermatitis. *J. Invest. Dermatol.,* **64,** 401–5

21. Ford, G. P., Farr, P. M., Ive, F. A. & Shuster, S. (1984). The response of seborrhoeic dermatitis to ketoconazole. *Br. J. Dermatol.,* **III Supp. 26,** 25

22. Farthing, C. F., Staughton, R. C. D. & Roland-Payne, C. M. E. (1985). Skin disease in homosexual patients with acquired immunodeficiency syndrome (AIDS) and lesser forms of human T cell leukaemia virus (HTLV-III) disease. *Clin. Exp. Dermatol.,* **10,** 3–12

23. Johnson, T. M., Duvic, M., Rapini, R. P. & Rios, A. (1985). AIDS exacerbates psoriasis. *N. Engl. J. Med.,* **313,** 1415

24. Farthing, C. F., Brown, S. E., Staughton, R. C. D., Cream, J. J. & Muhlemann, M. F. (1986). *A Colour Atlas of AIDS.* (Wolfe Medical Publications)

25. Chernosky, M. E. & Finley, V. K. (1985). Yellow nail syndrome in acquired

immunodeficiency disease. *J. Am. Acad. Dermatol.,* **13,** 731–6

26. Schwartz, B. K. & Clendenning, W. E. (1986). Pyoderma gangrenosum in a patient with HTLV antibody. *Arch. Dermatol.,* **122,** 508–9

27. Soeprono, F. F. & Schinella, R. A. (1986). Eosinophilic pustular folliculitis in patients with acquired immunodeficiency syndrome. *J. Am. Acad. Dermatol.,* **14,** 1020–2

28. Abramson, S. B., Odajynk, C. M., Grieco, A. J., Weissman, G. & Rosenstein, A. (1985). Hyperalgesic pseudothrombophlebitis. New syndrome in male homosexuals. *Am. J. Med.,* **78,** 317–20.

2

LIGHT ERUPTIONS

J. L. M. HAWK

Light-sensitivity eruptions, or photodermatoses, are common and often disabling skin diseases, frequently presenting problems of diagnosis and treatment. They are characterized by abnormal cutaneous reactions to ultraviolet (UV) and visible radiation but mechanistic details are usually uncertain. However, correct diagnosis is important to enable effective management.

UV and visible radiation, 100–400 and 400–800 nm in wavelength respectively, form part of the electromagnetic spectrum from sun and other light sources, terrestrial sunlight containing these wavelengths above about 290 nm as well as much heat. This radiation is made up of photon energy packets determined by wavelength and absorbed only by specific molecules capable of accepting such energy. The energetic molecules may then initiate chemical activity leading to ultimately observable effects, such as weathering of paintwork or the clinical features of a light eruption. Thus, in the latter, there is always UV or visible light absorption in the skin by a molecular photosensitizer, usually unidentified, before the events leading to the eruption.

UV radiation is made up of three wavebands of slightly varying biological effect. UVC (100–280 nm), not in terrestrial sunlight or most artificial radiation; UVB (280–315 nm), which is in sunlight and artificial radiation from equipment such as sunlamps, sunbeds and arc welding equipment and acutely induces cutaneous sunburn, tanning and many light eruptions and chronic ageing and cancer; and UVA (315–400 nm), which is in sunlight and artificial radiation from sunbed, psoralen photochemotherapy (PUVA) and white fluorescent lamps and also induces erythema and tanning (at about 1000 times greater doses than UVB), many light eruptions and, very likely, degenerative changes and cancer.

Light eruptions are induced only by skin exposure to UV or visible radiation and, in the absence of knowledge of pathogenesis and specific therapy, restriction of such exposure may be the only effective treatment. This may entail only avoidance of sunny holidays or else complete shunning of all light exposure, but knowledge of the physical behaviour of radiation as described below usually permits a reasonable patient lifestyle.

Solar UV, particularly UVB, intensity is greatest when atmospheric transit is shortest, around the solar midsummer zenith, notably at low latitudes and high altitudes, sunburn in fair subjects at such times occurring in 20 minutes or less. The radiation is also much less attenuated by cloud and haze than is heat and visible light, scanty shade from sun and cooling breeze giving little protection. On the other hand, UV reflection from snow, sand, light-coloured surfaces and rippling water and scattering from blue sky add considerably to its intensity, and it is fairly readily transmitted through water. Thus UV, particularly UVB, intensity may be high in cool or shady conditions around midday in summer, and low in hot, sunny weather at other times. UVB is about 1000 times more erythemogenic than UVA so that although 100 times less intense around midday it burns about 10 times more. However, UVA remains strong for much longer so that UVA sensitive patients must always be wary. Patients sensitive to visible light, generally the shorter blue–green rather than longer orange–red wavelengths, are at risk in all daylight, but less at dawn, dusk, in heavy cloud or indoors, unless exposed to fluorescent lights, tungsten lamps being preferable; television screens have no effect.

Modern high-protection factor topical sunbarrier preparations or sunscreens[1] also much reduce skin UV, particularly UVB, exposure although in practice they often do not work as well as might be expected. However, they are very important in treatment of most patients. Sunscreens are *absorbent* or *reflectant,* the former usually vanishing lotions, creams or oils which absorb UV radiation and disperse it as harmless quantities of heat. Active absorbing compounds include para-aminobenzoic acid (PABA) and its esters, anthranilates, cinnamates, salicylates, benzophenones and dibenzoylmethanes. Effectiveness is usually mostly in the UVB range, although some compounds, especially the latter, are also moderately useful against UVA. Reflectant compounds reflect radiation, being relatively effective against UVA and visible as well as UVB, and include the mixture of 25% titanium dioxide and 8% burnt sugar in aqueous cream, and proprietary camouflage preparations containing titanium dioxide or white Compound Zinc Paste BP.

To be useful, a sunscreen must be active against the wavelengths responsible for a light eruption, cosmetically acceptable and free of adverse effects. Sunscreen efficacy is denoted by the sun protection factor (SPF), which describes the increase in exposure before the onset of a given effect, usually sunburn – values ranging up to about 20 for very effective preparations. High SPF absorbent preparations are most useful for UVB- and moderately UVA-sensitive conditions, while reflectant preparations are most likely to help marked UVA or visible light sensitivity. Careful, regular application to exposed areas every hour or so is necessary for greatest efficiency, although some compounds, especially octyldimethyl PABA and PABA, are very resistant to removal by washing or exercise. Absorbent lotions are convenient and pleasant for unaffected skin protection, but often irritating or drying on rash, for which creams or oils are better. Some absorbent preparations contain small amounts of reflectant material such as titanium dioxide for better UVA protection, with only slight reduction in cosmetic acceptability. The fully reflectant compounds are generally coloured, messy and easily removed, and apart from the camouflage compounds for occasional female patients and zinc paste for limited use on sensitive areas such as lips and nose, they are used only as a last resort for extremely UVA- and visible light-sensitive patients. Preparations of low sensitizing potential are preferable for eczematous photosensitivity and necessary if contact or photocontact sensitivity occurs. Other adverse effects include relatively common transient, mild irritation particularly on broken skin, staining of clothing and other objects with PABA preparations, contact and photocontact dermatitis and acute inflammatory photoreactions. These general measures are helpful for many light eruptions but specific treatments discussed below are often more convenient and effective.

The light eruptions are:

1. Idiopathic photodermatoses

    (a) Polymorphic light eruption

    (b) Actinic prurigo

    (c) Chronic actinic dermatitis (a syndrome including actinic reticuloid, photosensitive eczema, and the photosensitivity dermatitis and actinic reticuloid (PD/AR) syndrome, and similar to some interpretations of persistent light reaction)

    (d) Solar urticaria

    (e) Hydroa vacciniforme

2. Metabolic photodermatoses

    (a) The porphyrias

        (i) Hepatic porphyrias

            Porphyria cutanea tarda
            Variegate porphyria
            Hereditary coproporphyria

        (ii) Erythropoietic porphyrias
            Congenital erythropoietic porphyria (Günther's disease)
            Erythropoietic protoporphyria

    (b) Xeroderma pigmentosum and other genodermatoses

3. Drug and chemical photosensitivity

4. UV-exacerbated dermatoses.

IDIOPATHIC PHOTODERMATOSES

Polymorphic light eruption (PLE)

This very common, persistent disorder affects about 10% of the population in temperate climates, mostly young women[2] (Figure 2.1). Its aetiology is possibly immunological, but induction is dependent on

28

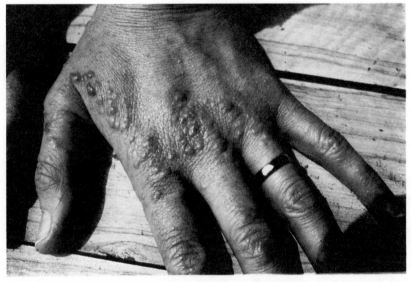

FIGURE 2.1 Polymorphic light eruption, macropapular variant: papules on backs of hands

exposure to summer or snow-reflected sunlight or solar simulated radiation, other artificial sources generally being ineffective.

The eruption develops some hours after minutes, hours or rarely up to two days of exposure, in black or white subjects, fading after hours, days or sometimes with continuing exposure, weeks. Characteristically and predominantly affected are symmetrically exposed areas of nose, malar regions of cheeks and chin, sides and back of neck, V of chest, backs of hands and dorsolateral aspects of arms, other exposed areas also being frequently affected, with sharp cut-off where clothing prevents UV penetration. Frequently in any patient, specific, often normally exposed areas, such as the face and backs of hands are not affected. Micropapular, pinhead-sized, confluent, erythematous, whitish or yellowish papules on an erythematous background may develop or macropapular, discrete, 2–3 mm flat or rounded, clustered lesions on normal skin may occur. In some patients there may be vesicles, confluent plaques, very rarely irritation without rash, and particularly on the face confluent erythema and swelling. Eczema-

29

tous PLE described in the USA is not generally recognized in the UK and may be mild chronic actinic dermatitis.

Solar urticaria is distinguished from PLE by its appearance within 5–10 minutes of exposure, persistence for only an hour or two after covering up and wealing. Actinic prurigo, very likely a variant of PLE, usually affects children with persistent excoriated papules of exposed sites, sometimes in association with typical PLE. Erythropoietic porphyria (EPP) is characterized by the onset of painful tingling within minutes of exposure and elevation of red blood cell protoporphyrin concentration. Sunlight-induced erythema multiforme is distinguished by histology. UV-exacerbated atopic and seborrhoeic eczemas differ in morphology and distribution.

Diagnosis is predominantly on history and clinical appearance if eruption is present. Blood antinuclear factor, Ro and La titres and porphyrin screening of blood, urine and stool exclude lupus erythematosus and porphyria. Histology shows focal epidermal spongiosis and dermal perivascular lymphocytic infiltrate. Irradiation skin tests with monochromator or broadband UVB and UVA sources occasionally demonstrate enhanced erythemal or papular responses to UVB or UVA, and solar simulated irradiation may sometimes induce the rash.

Treatment is by restriction of UV exposure and use of high SPF absorbent sunscreens, preferably with UVA efficacy. Low-dose psoralen photochemotherapy (PUVA) or UVB phototherapy 2–3 times weekly for 3–6 weeks before spring or vacation are very effective for patients who can attend a treatment centre[3]. Beta-carotene, chloroquine[4] and hydroxychloroquine[5] may rarely prevent, or in severe cases a 3–4 day course of oral prednisolone rapidly abate, the eruption.

Actinic prurigo

This disorder (Figure 2.2), possibly a persistent, excoriated PLE variant, usually affects children until adolescence, and occasionally adults, all predominantly female, while adult American Indians suffer a very similar condition.

The disease is worse in summer and may clear completely in winter, a variation often unnoticed by the patient, and may flare after sun

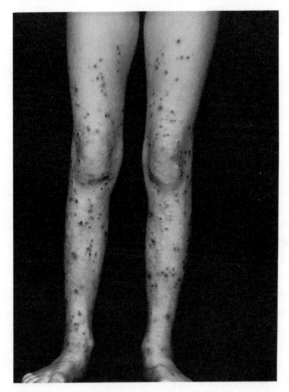

FIGURE 2.2   Actinic prurigo: excoriated papules on legs, more profuse distally

exposure, sometimes as typical PLE. There are excoriated, sometimes crusted papules or nodules on V of chest, upper back, face and limbs, more profuse distally, often with shallow, linear, punctate or irregular flat scars on the face and forehead, and sparing under the hair fringe. Sacrum and buttocks are also affected on occasions.

Atopic eczema and prurigo, insect bites, prurigo nodularis, occasionally scabies and, because of the facial scarring, erythropoietic protoporphyria must be differentiated. Diagnosis in mild cases may be difficult and is principally by history and clinical appearance. Monochromator tests sometimes show enhanced erythemal or papular responses, both UVB and UVA probably contributing to the eruption.

Treatment is by restriction of UV exposure and use of high SPF

31

absorbent sunscreens. Low dose PUVA and UVB phototherapy as for PLE may be of some effect, but for severe cases, intermittent courses of low dose thalidomide 50–100 mg or less daily are very effective[6] although teratogenicity and tendency to induce peripheral neuropathy necessitate extreme care in its use.

Chronic actinic dermatitis (CAD)[7]

This includes the severe actinic reticuloid variant[8], the milder photosensitive eczema[9], and the photosensitivity dermatitis and actinic reticuloid (PD/AR) syndrome[10]. CAD is a not uncommon, often severely incapacitating form of eczematous photosensitivity largely affecting middle-aged and elderly men (Figures 2.3, 2.4). Its cause is unknown but photosensitized activation of exogenous or endogenous allergens may be important, some instances of allergic photosensitivity to chemicals and drugs being clinically indistinguishable. Musk ambrette in toilet preparations has been particularly implicated[11]. A causal relationship has also been suggested with allergic contact sensitivity particularly to airborne allergens such as Compositae plant oleoresins, especially chrysanthemum, phosphorus sesquisulphide and colophony but also rubber, metals and topical applications by an as yet poorly understood mechanism[12], but perhaps more likely contact sensitivity to such sensitizers merely exacerbates already eczematous skin.

Black and white subjects sometimes with history of other eczema may be affected, worse in summer and after sun exposure, often not recognized by patients. Widespread eczema, often lichenified, follicular or associated with infiltrated, erythematous, shiny papules or plaques affects exposed skin of the face, scalp, back and sides of the neck, V of chest and backs of arms and hands, sometimes with spared, exposed or affected, covered areas. Skin creases accentuated by the infiltration and skin folds are spared in their depths on forehead, face, groins, fingerwebs, and upper eyelids. Palmar and plantar eczema may occur. Eyebrows and eyelashes may be broken or lost. Irregular areas of pigmentation are common. Purpura of affected sites may be present. In severe cases there may be generalized erythroderma, not always more marked on exposed sites. Patients may be severely dis-

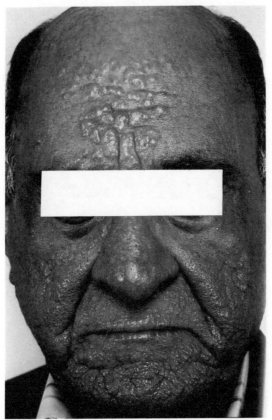

FIGURE 2.3 Chronic actinic dermatitis: actinic reticuloid variant with infiltrated papules and plaques, and sparing of some light exposed areas

abled and become depressed. There is occasional gradual spontaneous remission.

CAD must be differentiated from airborne contact dermatitis unassociated with light sensitivity by the distribution of the rash, and in patients with infiltrated plaques from mycosis fungoides, the histology of which may be virtually indistinguishable. The severe light sensitivity of CAD distinguishes, although mycosis fungoides may occasionally be associated with mild light sensitivity[13]. Erythrodermic CAD resembles the Sézary syndrome, large numbers of circulating Sézary cells being present in both[14], but the marked light sensitivity of CAD

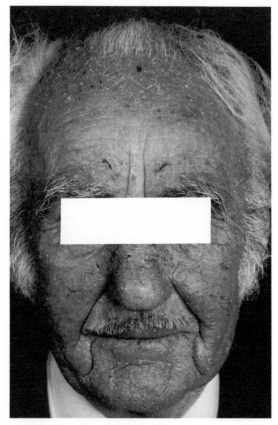

FIGURE 2.4   Chronic actinic dermatitis: photosensitive eczema variant with sparing of upper eyelids.

again differentiates. Erythrodermic CAD must also be distinguished from other non-Sézary forms of erythroderma.

Irradiation skin tests are essential to establish diagnosis and to determine the causative wavelengths to facilitate treatment. Lower than normal radiation doses for erythema and swelling occur in the UVB, often extending to UVA and occasionally visible light wavelengths as well. Irradiation tests may sometimes remain normal for months after disease onset and should be repeated if clinical suspicion of CAD persists. Skin biopsy shows eczematous changes with deep dermal lymphohistiocytic infiltrate and in infiltrated areas epidermal cellular invasion with Pautrier-like epidermal cell collections suggesting mycosis fungoides. Patch tests often demonstrate reactions to a variety of allergens such as airborne plant sensitizers and sunscreen constituents, not always of definite clinical importance. Photopatch tests may demonstrate a photosensitizer, such as sunscreen constituent, exacerbating CAD or primarily inducing clinically identical photocontact dermatitis.

Restriction or in severe cases virtual avoidance of radiation exposure is necessary. Commercially available plastic film blinds filter most UV and short visible radiation to give excellent skin protection while allowing reasonable yellowish illumination. Sunscreens are very useful although seldom totally effective, the most cosmetically acceptable absorbent type unfortunately useful in UVB- and short wavelength UVA-sensitive CAD only, and the messy, coloured reflectant and time-consuming camouflage preparations most suitable but unpopular for visible light-sensitive CAD, combined absorbent/reflectant preparations generally being used as a compromise instead.

Orally administered azathioprine is very effective in the majority of CAD patients in a dose of about 2 mg/kg/day for up to several months, with gradual onset of remission for months to years[15]. Red, white and platelet cell counts and liver function should be monitored monthly throughout treatment, while adverse gastrointestinal effects such as pain, nausea and diarrhoea in some patients may necessitate termination of therapy. If azathioprine is unsuccessful, PUVA therapy two to three times weekly for weeks to months with oral and topical steroid cover, if necessary, may induce clearing, low initial UVA doses $(0.25–0.5 \, \text{J/cm}^2)$ being advisable until the eruption begins to settle[16]. Some patients cannot tolerate the therapy.

Solar urticaria (SU)

This rare disorder (Figure 2.5) of all age groups and both sexes is of unknown cause, although apparently immunologically based in some [17]. Any waveband in the UV or visible spectrum, relatively constant for a given patient, may evoke wealing. Tingling develops five to ten minutes after exposure on irradiated sites, except often regularly uncovered areas such as face and backs of hands, followed

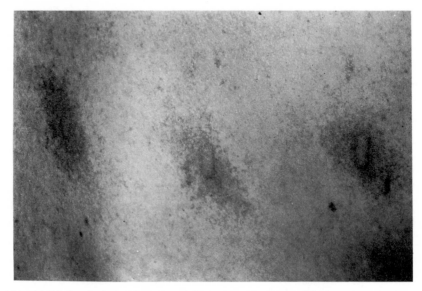

FIGURE 2.5   Solar urticaria: weals induced by monochromatic irradiation

rapidly by erythema and weal formation, often confluent with a sharp demarcation line at clothing, the eruption abating within one to two hours of covering up. Temporary lack of reactivity may occur if exposure is repeated within up to 24 hours. PLE, occasionally systemic lupus erythematosus, very rarely porphyria, particularly erythro-poietic protoporphyria, and photosensitivity to topically applied agents such as tar, pitch and dyes may be associated with SU.

SU may be confused with PLE because of somewhat similar time course, but appears much sooner and settles more rapidly, and with other photodermatoses of early onset such as lupus erythematosus and drug or chemical photosensitivity. SU is best diagnosed by solar or artificial induction of lesions, although the latter is not always effective. Monochromatic irradiation tests define action spectrum to aid disease classification and treatment.

UVB-sensitive SU may respond to absorbent high SPF sunscreen use and restricted radiation exposure. The newer non-sedative H_1 antihistamines, terfenadine and astemizole, slightly more effective with the H_2 agent, cimetidine[18], give some protection in high doses[19]. Regular exposure to the inducing wavelengths from sunlight or arti-

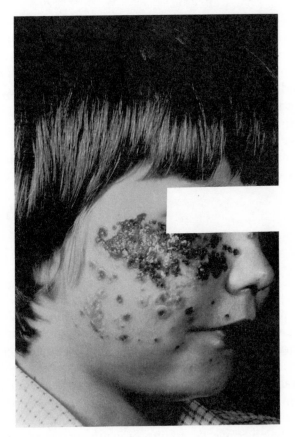

FIGURE 2.6 Hydroa vacciniforme: vesicles, some umbilicated, with crusting on face (kindly contributed by Dr Margaret Price)

ficial sources may help[20] and PUVA is sometimes effective[21]. However, SU remains a therapeutic problem.

Hydroa vacciniforme (HV)[22]

This very rare, recurrent eruption of unknown aetiology affects mainly children and young adults (Figure 2.6), UVA appearing responsible in most patients. Within hours of summer sun exposure, particularly on face and backs of hands, clusters of 2–3 mm erythematous macules develop into discrete or confluent vesicles which umbilicate over a day or so, scab and heal into pitted, varioliform scars. The condition must be distinguished from PLE, actinic prurigo, herpes simplex and hepatic porphyria, by the history, severe scarring and histology. Diagnosis is clinical and histological, vesicle biopsy showing mid-epidermal necrosis and dermal leucocytic infiltrate. UV restriction and sun-screens giving UVA protection are helpful, and oral chloroquine, PUVA and UVB phototherapy have been used with occasional success. Remission may occur during adolescence or the disorder may persist into adult life.

METABOLIC PHOTODERMATOSES

The hepatic porphyrias

Porphyria cutanea tarda (PCT)

This not uncommon disorder principally of the middle-aged and elderly (Figure 2.7) may be the autosomal dominant familial form, or the sporadic consequent on effects of consumed hepatotoxins, particularly alcohol, oestrogens or polyhalogenated hydrocarbons such as hexachlorobenzene. Both types are associated with a deficiency of the haem biosynthetic enzyme uroporphyrinogen decarboxylase, systemic in the familial and hepatic only in the sporadic, excess uropor-phyrinogen being converted to photosensitizing uroporphyrin in skin leading to the clinical abnormalities[23].

Exposed skin, more in summer, of backs of hands and occasionally forehead, face and scalp very readily forms erosions and bullae after minor injury, often with infection, before crusting and healing with superficial scarring. There may also be milia, hypertrichosis, irregular pigmentation, scarring alopecia and reversible scleroderma-like changes of exposed sites. Alcohol consumption is often excessive. Diabetes mellitus, lupus erythematosus and hepatoma are very rarely associated.

PCT is differentiated from variegate porphyria and hereditary coproporphyria by porphyrin assay of urine, stool and blood. Epi-dermolysis bullosa acquisita and occasionally bullous amyloidosis may have similar clinical and histological appearance, while other

38

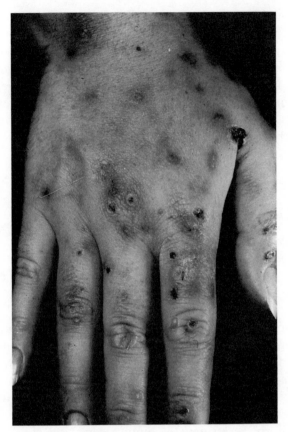

FIGURE 2.7   Porphyria cutanea tarda: erosions and crusting on back of hands

blistering disorders such as pemphigus, pemphigoid and dermatitis herpetiformis are clinically and histologically different; normal porphyrin biochemistry and immunofluorescent findings differentiate. PCT occasionally resembles superficial infection, scabies or excoriations but porphyrin assay distinguishes.

Urinary uroporphyrin and to lesser extent coproporphyrin concentrations are elevated in PCT, stool porphyrins may be slightly raised or normal and isocoproporphyrin may be present, while red blood cell porphyrins are normal. Serum liver transaminase, iron and porphyrin and blood iron and haemoglobin concentrations are often raised. Liver biopsy may be normal or show fatty infiltration or cirrhosis. Cutaneous irradiation tests often show abnormal erythematous, petechial or urticarial responses around 400–600 nm.

Avoidance of ethyl alcohol, oestrogens, iron and other hepatotoxins is essential in PCT therapy and may lead alone to clinical and biochemical cure. Otherwise, 500 ml venesection every 2 weeks or so for 3–6 months or, more conveniently, low dose oral chloroquine 125 mg twice weekly for 6–12 months are safe and effective. Relapse may occur in months to years requiring further treatment[24].

Variegate porphyria (VP)

This relatively rare autosomal dominant porphyria, particularly affecting South African whites, usually has onset around adolescence and is associated with protoporphyrinogen oxidase haem biosynthetic enzyme deficiency and excessive tissue accumulation of coproporphyrin.

Skin abnormalities occur as in PCT and systemic attacks as in acute intermittent porphyria with abdominal pain, paralysis, mania or coma, sometimes fatal. Latent cases are common. Many drugs may precipitate attacks, relatively few being safe[25].

Differential diagnosis of the skin abnormalities is as for PCT and of the systemic crises as for acute intermittent porphyria. Diagnosis is by porphyrin assessment in blood, urine and stool, there being stool protoporphyrin more than coproporphyrin increase, and urinary coproporphyrin more than uroporphyrin increase, with raised aminolaevulinic acid and porphobilinogen during systemic attacks. In difficult cases so called porphyrin X in stool, and plasma 624 nm fluorescence are characteristic of VP. Irradiation skin tests may reveal abnormalities at 400–600 nm.

Treatment is avoidance of precipitating drugs, alcohol and metabolic stresses. Systemic attacks may respond to 20% intravenous laevulose, intravenous haematin or more recently and safely haem arginate[26]; other therapies for specific complications may be required.

VP persists throughout life but may not cause problems with avoidance of precipitating factors, or continuing cutaneous symptoms and occasional systemic crises may occur.

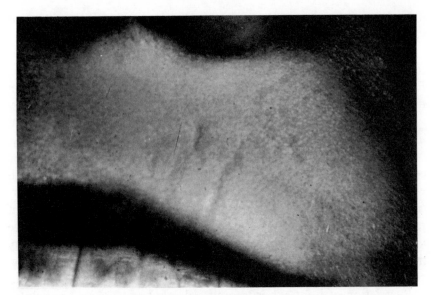

FIGURE 2.8   Erythropoietic protoporphyria: scars radiating from lips

Hereditary coproporphyria (HC)

This extremely rare autosomal dominant condition clinically resembling VP is associated with coproporphyrinogen oxidase enzyme deficiency, with markedly raised stool and urinary corproporphyrin concentrations. Differential diagnosis and treatment are as for VP, with somewhat better prognosis, systemic attacks being less easily provoked.

Erythropoietic protoporphyria (EPP)

This relatively common porphyria of dominant inheritance with usual childhood onset has ferrochelatase enzyme deficiency and excessive red blood cell and other tissue protoporphyrin, including skin (Figure 2.8).

Painful, invisible, skin irritation after minutes' summer sun exposure, worse if windy, is followed after hours' continuing exposure by swelling persisting for several days. Acute purpura, erythema, wealing and vesicles occur rarely.

Chronic signs are commonly waxy, linear, punctate or irregular flat scars on face or nose. Radial furrows may extend from lip margins. Exposed skin may have coarse, dry texture. Knuckle skin is often thickened with skin marking accentuation following infiltration by type IV basement membrane collagen[27]. Porphyrin gallstones and fatal liver failure are rare. SU, drug and chemical induced photosensitivity, rarely PLE and occasionally the light-exacerbated dermatoses may be confused with EPP, but markedly raised red blood cell protoporphyrin with sometimes moderate stool increase distinguishes. Urinary porphyrins are not raised except in terminal hepatic failure. Transient red blood cell fluorescence may be observed under the fluorescence microscope. Hepatic transaminase blood levels are occasionally minimally raised. Skin irradiation at 400–600 nm may induce tingling, erythema, purpura, pigmentation or rarely wealing.

Restriction of light exposure and reflectant sunscreens are helpful in treatment, although the latter are too unsightly for regular use. Beta-carotene usually combined with canthaxanthin, up to 200 mg daily, in summer has improved many patients in uncontrolled studies, although recent reports of possible defective dark vision from retinal canthaxanthin deposits have indicated the need for cautious use. EPP is lifelong, often with gradual improvement in light tolerance.

Xeroderma pigmentosum and other genodermatoses

Xeroderma pigmentosum (XP)[28] (Figure 2.9) is rare, autosomal recessive and characterized often by easy, severe sunburning, generally first noted in infancy, and usually by early onset of degenerative eye changes and cutaneous ageing and cancer, fatal without treatment, all resulting from defective repair of UVB-induced nuclear DNA damage. There are nine genetic complementation groups, A to I, of abnormal excision repair, A, C and D most common, and one, XP variant, of post-replication repair.

Clinical features on exposed areas are easy sunburning (commonly groups A and D), gradually increasing dryness, freckling, telangiectasia and squamous, basal and melanocarcinomas. Certain com-

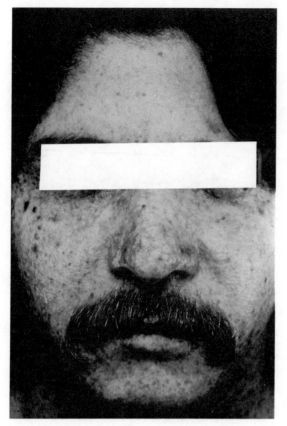

FIGURE 2.9   Xeroderma pigmentosum: degenerative changes on facial skin

plementation groups are associated with only mild clinical features and others (particularly A, D and G) with severe progressive neuro-logical and mental deficiency.

Diagnosis is by clinical assessment, irradiation skin tests often showing enhanced, delayed erythemal responses to UVB and by showing reduced DNA repair by cultured fibroblasts. The com-plementation group is that group whose cells fused with patient cells do not abolish the repair defect.

Treatment is by restriction of UV exposure and high SPF sunscreen use, which may slow progression. There is no neurological defect

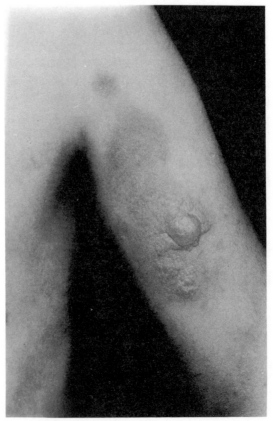

FIGURE 2.10 Drug and chemical photosensitivity: phytophoto-dermatitis from contact with psoralen-containing plants

treatment. Prenatal diagnosis is possible if severe foetal XP is suspected.

Bloom's, Cockayne's and the Rothmund–Thomson syndromes are very rare photosensitive genodermatoses associated with multiple congenital defects and impaired or shortened patient lives.

DRUG AND CHEMICAL PHOTOSENSITIVITY

This is from exposure to plant, therapeutic, cosmetic or industrial photosensitizing agents, particularly the first three (Figure 2.10). They are generally organic, planar, cyclic or long-chain compounds with alternating single and double bonds and absorb UVA within skin to give various acute inflammatory or immunologically mediated clinical consequences.

Several clinical reactions are possible. Some contact photosensitizers such as tar, pitch, dyes and systemic agents such as benoxaprofen and EPP porphyrins regularly cause variable, painful, skin irritation within minutes of exposure often followed by erythema, oedema, vesiculation or rarely wealing. Some systemic photosensitizers such as frusemide, nalidixic acid and naproxen and PCT, VP, and HC porphyrins occasionally cause skin fragility, subepidermal bullae, crusting, superficial scarring and milia. Some contact and systemic photosensitizers, particularly the musk ambrette fragrance and fixative in many cosmetics and toiletries and the previously important halogenated salicylanilides rarely lead to eczema of uncovered areas which may progress to resemble CAD. Oral and topical photosensitizers have been listed[29].

SU may resemble drug and chemical photosensitivity because of tingling and wealing, but without photosensitizer. EPP also causes tingling, occasional erythema and rare wealing, but is distinguished by raised red blood cell protoporphyrin. Lupus erythematosus, particularly systemic, is associated with erythema of exposed sites but distinguished by immunological abnormality. Airborne contact dermatitis and CAD resemble eczematous drug and chemical photosensitivity, but patch, photopatch and irradiation tests lead to diagnosis. Sunburn may resemble acute inflammatory drug and chemical photosensitivity but is less marked for similar exposure.

Irradiation skin tests from monochromatic or other artificial sources in chemical and drug photosensitivity are usually normal but may elicit abnormal irritation, erythema, wealing or papules with UVA or rarely UVB or visible irradiation. Photopatch tests to topical photosensitizers may be positive or commonly negative. Clinical evaluation is most important in diagnosis.

Photosensitizer avoidance is the most effective treatment, light restriction being necessary if this is impossible. Only reflectant sunscreens are likely to be useful since UVA is generally responsible for the photosensitivity. Chronic eczematous photosensitivity may be slow to improve even after photosensitizer removal, necessitating CAD treatment.

Acute photosensitivity to oral or topical agents usually resolves within a day or two of photosensitizer removal but widespread eczematous syndromes may persist for months, perhaps because of persisting exposure to minute quantities of photosensitizer, or perhaps with total photosensitizer avoidance by an unknown mechanism, called persistent light reaction.

UV-EXACERBATED DERMATOSES

Dermatoses of non-photosensitive aetiology may be precipitated or aggravated in some patients by UV exposure, although not affected or improved in others. These include rosacea, atopic eczema, psoriasis, seborrhoeic eczema, erythema multiforme, herpes simplex, lupus erythematosus (discoid and systemic), lichen planus, Darier's disease, pemphigus foliaceus and pemphigus erythematosus, the first four also sometimes improved by exposure. UVB exposure is usually responsible but mechanisms are generally unknown. Exposed areas or sites of predilection of the condition are affected. Diagnosis is as for the underlying condition with a story of sunlight exacerbation. However, confusion is possible with short-lived disorders such as erythema multiforme and mild atopic eczema with PLE and of erythemas such as lupus erythematosus with EPP, SU and drug and chemical photosensitivity. Cutaneous irradiation and other tests are generally normal. Treatment is restriction of UVB exposure, sunscreen use and treatment of the underlying dermatosis.

References

1. Murphy, G. M. and Hawk, J. L. M., (1986). Sunscreens (Editorial). *J. R. Soc. Med.*, **79**, 254–6
2. Morison, W. L. and Stern, R. S. (1982). Polymorphous light eruption: a common reaction uncommonly recognised. *Acta Derm. Venereol.*, **62**, 237–40
3. Murphy, G. M., Logan, R. A., Lovell, C. R., Morris, R. W., Hawk, J. L. M. and Magnus, I. A. (1987). Prophylactic PUVA and UVB therapy in polymorphic light eruption – a controlled trial. *Br. J. Dermatol.*, **116**, 531–8

4. Corbett, M. F., Hawk, J. L. M., Herxheimer, A. and Magnus, I. A. (1982). Controlled therapeutic trials in polymorphic light eruption. *Br. J. Dermatol.*, **107**, 571–81

5. Murphy, G. M., Hawk., J. L. M. and Magnus, I. A. (1987). Hydroxychloroquine in polymorphic light eruption: a controlled trial with drug and visual sensitivity monitoring. *Br. J. Dermatol.*, **116**, 379–86

6. Lovell, C. R., Hawk, J. L. M., Calnan, C. D. and Magnus, I. A. (1983). Thalidomide in actinic prurigo. *Br. J. Dermatol.*, **108**, 467–71

7. Hawk, J. L. M. and Magnus, I. A. (1979). Chronic actinic dermatitis – an idiopathic photosensitivity syndrome including actinic reticuloid and photosensitive eczema. *Br. J. Dermatol.*, **101 (Suppl. 17)**, 24

8. Ive, F. A., Magnus, I. A., Warin, R. P. and Wilson Jones, E. (1969). Actinic reticuloid; a chronic dermatosis associated with severe photosensitivity and the histological resemblance to lymphoma. *Br. J. Dermatol.*, **81**, 469–85

9. Ramsay, C. A. and Kobza-Black, A. (1973). Photosensitive eczema. *Trans. St John's Hospital Dermatol. Soc.*, **59**, 152–8

10. Frain-Bell, W., Lakshmipathi, J. Rogers, J. and Willock, J. (1974). The syndrome of chronic photosensitivity dermatitis and actinic reticuloid. *Br. J. Dermatol.*, **91**, 617–34

11. Wojnarowska F. and Calnan, C. D. (1986). Contact and photocontact allergy to musk ambrette. *Br. J. Dermatol.*, **114**, 667–75

12. Frain-Bell, W. and Johnson, B. E. (1979). Contact allergic sensitivity to plants and the photosensitivity dermatitis and actinic reticuloid syndrome. *Br. J. Dermatol.*, **101**, 503–12

13. Volden, G. and Thune, P. O. (1977). Light sensitivity in mycosis fungoides. *Br. J. Dermatol.* **97**, 279–84.

14. Neild, V. S., Hawk, J. L. M., Eady, R. A. J. and Cream, J. J. (1982). Actinic reticuloid with Sézary cells. *Clin. Exp. Dermatol.*, **7**, 143–8

15. Leigh, I. M. and Hawk, J. L. M. (1984). Treatment of chronic actinic dermatitis with azathioprine. *Br. J. Dermatol.*, **110**, 691–5

16. Hindson, C., Spiro, J. and Downey, A. (1985). PUVA therapy of chronic actinic dermatitis. *Br. J. Dermatol.*, **113**, 157–60

17. Harber, L. C., Holloway, R. M., Wheatley, V. R. and Baer, R. L. (1963). Immunologic and biophysical studies in solar urticaria. *J. Invest. Dermatol.*, **41**, 439–43

18. Michell, P., Hawk, J. L. M., Shafrir, A., Corbett, M. F. and Magnus, I. A. (1980). Assessing the treatment of solar urticaria. The dose response as a quantifying response. *Dermatologica*, **160**, 198–207

19. Murphy, G. M. and Hawk, J. L. M. (1987). Solar urticaria with alteration of action spectrum. *Clin. Exp. Dermatol.* (in press)

20. Ramsay, C. A. (1977). Solar urticaria treatment by inducing tolerance to artificial radiation and natural light. *Arch. Dermatol.*, **113**, 1222–5

21. Parrish, J. A., Jaenicke, K. F., Morison, W. L., Momtaz, K. and Shea, C. (1982). Solar urticaria: treatment with PUVA and mediator inhibitors. *Br. J. Dermatol.*, **106**, 575–80

22. Sonnex, T. S. and Hawk, J. L. M. (1987). Hydroa vacciniforme, a review of ten cases. *Br. J. Dermatol.* (in press)

23. Elder, G. H., Sheppard, D. M., Salemanca, R. E. and Olmos, A. (1980). Identification of two types of porphyria cutanea tarda by measurements of erythrocytic uroporphyrinogen decarboxylase. *Clin. Sci.*, **58**, 477–84

47

24. Ashton, R. E., Hawk, J. L. M. and Magnus, I. A. (1984). Low-dose oral chloro-quine in the treatment of porphyria cutanea tarda. *Br. J. Dermatol.*, **111,** 609–13
25. Moore, M. R. and Disler, P. B. (1983). Drug-induction of the acute porphyrias. *Adverse Drug React. Acute Poisoning Rev.*, **2,** 149–89
26. Mustajoki, P., Tenhunen, R., Tokola, O. and Gothoni, G. (1986). Haem arginate in the treatment of acute hepatic porphyrias. *Br. Med. J.*, **293,** 538–9
27. Murphy, G. M., Hawk, J. L. M. and Magnus, I. A. (1985). Late-onset erythro-poietic protoporphyria with unusual cutaneous features. *Arch. Dermatol.*, **121,** 1309–12
28. Pawsey, S. A., Magnus, I. A., Ramsay, C. A., Benson, P. F. and Giannelli, F. (1979). Clinical, genetic and DNA repair studies on a consecutive series of patients with xeroderma pigmentosum. *Q. J. Med.*, **48,** 179–210
29. Hawk, J. L. M. (1984). Photosensitising agents used in the United Kingdom. *Clin. Exp. Dermatol.*, **9,** 300–2

3
ASPECTS OF ITCHING

R. M. GRAHAM

INTRODUCTION

An itch is an uncomfortable non-adapting cutaneous sensation, which provokes the desire to scratch or rub. It is the principal presenting symptom in dermatology patients. Unfortunately, as a cutaneous symptom it tends to be poorly localized. Pruritus has been reported[1] as the prime cause of 2.8% of general practice consultations.

The crucial aspect in the management of pruritus is an accurate diagnosis of its aetiology; when a condition has been labelled as idiopathic then all reasonable avenues should have been explored to exclude cutaneous or systemic disease. The therapeutic modalities available to manage idiopathic pruritus are so limited that the patient inappropriately confined to this group is dealt a great disservice, if not a fatal blow, in the case of underlying malignancy.

ANATOMY AND PHYSIOLOGY

Itch and pain are so closely allied that the former is often considered as a sub-threshold of the latter. The itch receptor is a free unmyelinated nerve ending, situated in close proximity to the dermo–epidermal junction. These receptors occur in the mucous membranes and cornea as well as the skin, but it is doubtful whether the buccal and nasal mucosae can truly exhibit the itch sensation. The cornea, however, certainly can[2] and is a potential site for localized itching to occur. Itch receptors respond to physical stimuli such as, heat, electricity and prick, together with chemical stimuli, e.g. histamine and kinins; they are therefore known as polymodal. Prostaglandins, however, do not directly cause stimulation, but as with dry skin may lower the threshold for itching to occur. Histamine is the archetypal peripheral mediator of pruritus; when introduced into the epidermis, it is usually accompanied by a wheal and flare response, but if higher doses are administered into the dermis, then the sensation of itch changes to pain. The effects of histamine are predominantly executed via H_1 receptors. However, there is an indirect action on other mediators such as substance P and prostaglandins; possibly other receptors are also involved[3]. Substance P and other peptides, e.g. bradykinin, are in themselves potent histamine releasers, the effects of which are counteracted by antihistamines. Kallikrein, a proteolytic enzyme, can cause marked pruritus, but this is not affected by antihistamine and does not produce a wheal and flare. The itching produced by *Mucuna pruriens,* alternatively known as cowhage, is also mediated by pathways other than histamine; this legume has, occasionally, been the cause of outbreaks of pruritus; analysis of the plant has revealed the presence of 5–hydrotryptamine[4].

Both poorly localized, persistent itch and dull pain are transmitted on unmyelinated C fibres, but there is evidence that they are carried on different populations of primary sensory neurones[5]. Spontaneous localized pricking itch, however, may be carried on myelinated A delta fibres[6]. Both these fibres enter the spinal cord via the dorsal horn, synapse, cross the midline and travel in the anterolateral spinothalamic tracts in close association with the pain fibres. In cases of transection of the tract, the modalities of both pain and itch are lost[7]. The ascending fibres relay in the substantia gelatinosa, then in the posterior lateral ventral nucleus of the thalamus and pass to the posterior central gyrus of the sensory cortex. It has been inferred that a central mechanism for itch also exists in the medulla and that these receptors respond to endogenous opioids[8]: enkephalins may therefore act at this level and other sites to modify the perception of itch. The central processes of itching are poorly understood; at a higher level conscious perception of itch may be modified by a variety of factors, particularly the psychological make-up of the individual, but distracting environmental and mental factors are also important.

HISTORY

A thorough personal and family history will save the clinician time and embarrassment, together with prevention of unnecessary patient investigation and suffering. A good approach is to start with the date, site and circumstances of onset, the subsequent distribution, include any associations and precipitating factors observed by the patient and conclude with the current situation. The occurrence of a similar problem in others is especially important with contagious conditions, such as scabies (Figure 3.1). An occupational history, e.g. work with fibreglass or other pruritogens may help with aetiology. Physical environmental factors such as high or low humidity and atmospheric dust may be relevant in the work place. Document any past history of skin or internal disease: a similar family history should also be taken, as diatheses are often inherited in skin disease.

Details of any foreign travel should be noted: onchocerciasis often presents with a generalized pruritus, as well as a non-specific rash. Tungiasis[9], by comparison, can cause localized itching, usually on the foot. Both conditions may follow travel to Central Africa or South America.

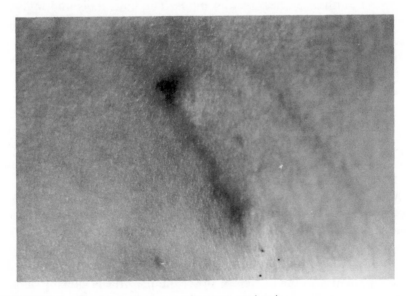

FIGURE 3.1   Scabietic burrow: close up on back

A drug history may be important not only in the use and abuse of opiate drugs, but also in allergic drug reactions, where itching can antedate the development of a rash and in the case of potentially cholestatic drugs, such as chlorpromazine, precede the development of jaundice. When treating patients with retinoids for disorders of keratinization, it is worth remembering that etretinate can also cause generalized pruritus[10].

EXAMINATION

It is imperative that the patient is fully undressed; obviously this should be tempered by common sense and be appropriate to the problem but it is common for vital skin signs to pass unnoticed by the patient. Careful inspection of the skin is required, particularly when excluding scabies, in which special attention should be paid to the interdigital spaces, feet, groin and axillae. In the case of the latter two sites, post-scabietic nodules may be the only sign of an infestation which has settled but has left the patient with persistent pruritus for up to a month after clearance of mites. The hair, nails and mucosal surfaces should not be forgotten as these may reflect both cutaneous and systemic disorders. Polished nails and broken hairs secondary to scratching may be a useful indication of the degree of irritation. Especially in fair-haired individuals, pediculosis may easily be missed; as well as examining scalp, pubic and axillary hair, clothing should be inspected for nits. In addition to localized itching and eczematous rashes, a more generalized, itchy pediculid[11] may occur. When no apparent abnormality is visible and infestations have been excluded ensure that asteatosis is not overlooked, as dry skin is a common cause of pruritus, particularly in the elderly.

With the exception of minor, localized, readily diagnosed causes of itching, examination of the skin should be followed by a complete medical examination of the systems; with particular attention to the lymph nodes and abdominal organs. During the history and examination it is helpful to make an assessment of the psychological state of the patient and the degree of upset the pruritus is causing, as this may influence diagnosis and management.

INVESTIGATION

The investigation of the 'itchy patient' should be adapted to suit that individuals' problem; this may be immediately obvious but is more often, at least initially, obscure. In general, cases can be divided into those due to primary skin disease and those secondary to systemic disorders. In either group the condition may be generalized or localized to a specific site or sites. A further category of idiopathic is unfortunately necessary and it is in this group that emotional and psychological factors may be more pertinent.

A good clinical algorithm for the investigation of a patient with generalized pruritus has been described by Champion[12]. A list of baseline investigations for unexplained pruritus is given in Table 3.1. This is predominantly applicable to the patient with generalized

TABLE 3.1 Baseline investigations for unexplained pruritus

Haemoglobin, full blood count, film and ESR
Blood urea and serum electrolytes
Liver function tests
Serum thyroxine, T_3 and free thyroxine index
Serum iron and total iron binding capacity
Plasma and urine, protein electrophoresis
Urine analysis for protein, sugar and microscopy
Chest X-ray

---

pruritus in the absence of primary skin lesions. However, one problem that even the experienced clinician may find difficult is the distinction between primary cutaneous changes and those secondary to prolonged scratching. This is highlighted by one of the commonest pruritic skin conditions, atopic eczema, in which the results of scratching, e.g. excoriations and lichenification, are the principal skin changes (Figures 3.2, 3.3). In these and many other circumstances, skin biopsy and histological analysis with or without immunofluorescent studies may prove helpful.

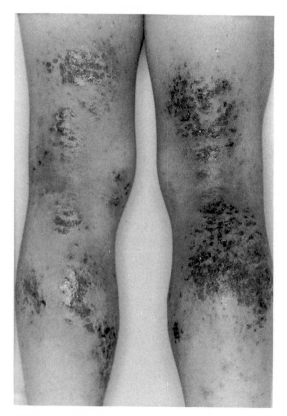

FIGURE 3.2   Excoriated atopic eczema

ITCHING AND PRIMARY SKIN DISEASE

A list of dermatoses that are commonly associated with itching is given in Table 3.2. It is not within the scope of this article to deal with

TABLE 3.2 Skin conditions associated with generalized itching

---

Endogenous eczema: atopic, discoid, seborrhoeic, varicose and asteatotic
Exogenous eczema: both irritant and allergic contact eczema
Urticaria, urticaria pigmentosa, mastocytosis and dermatographism
Psoriasis, pityriasis rosea, and lichen planus
Dermatitis herpetiformis and bullous pemphigoid
Insect bites, infections and infestations especially scabies and pediculosis.

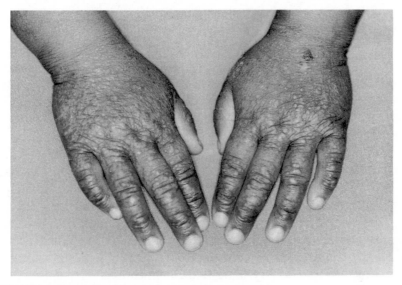

FIGURE 3.3   Lichenification in atopic eczema

each of these, but there are several important aspects which are worthy of mention.

Itching is a cardinal symptom in dermatological patients. However, its presence or absence should not be used to establish or exclude any diagnosis, rather it should be used as a pointer to direct a clinician to an avenue of diagnostic possibilities which require further substantiation. This is because patients may vary considerably in their degree of itching in response to similar and equally severe dermatoses. Furthermore, dermatoses which are painful when scratched, such as lichen planus, may lose their pruritic element, as pain can surpass itch in being appreciated by the conscious mind. It has been suggested that itching can elevate the pain threshold, via the effect of antidromic nerve impulses; this may explain why clearly painful excoriations can be self-inflicted, while the patient appears to be enjoying the scratch response to an itch[13]. Timing of intensity of itch has also been ascribed as a diagnostic pointer, particularly in scabies, with a nocturnal exacerbation. However, most pruritic eruptions are worst at night and this timing does not usefully serve to distinguish one from another. Care must also be taken with physical associations, e.g. water may precipitate aquagenic pruritus[14], but bathing can, if hot, exacerbate any itchy dermatosis and if cooling occurs, precipitation of cold urticaria or polycythaemia rubra vera may occur[15]. There appears to be a subset of aquagenic pruritus that affects elderly females with dry skin, in whom antihistamines tend to be unhelpful, but symptoms improve with hydrophobic ointments[14]; separation from asteatotic eczema therefore may prove difficult. Itching is the cardinal feature of atopic eczema, in which the skin changes are predominantly a reflection of the prolonged scratching. It has been observed that some Asian patients with generalized pruritus have an atopic diathesis without cutaneous evidence of such, perhaps accounting for their itching[16]. Both exogenous and endogenous types of eczema are itchy but the intensity varies considerably between the different forms. Juvenile plantar dermatosis is often thought to be non-itchy but itching occurs in at least 10% of cases, soreness perhaps overriding the itch sensation in many of the others. Dry skin often complicates eczema and exacerbates most cases of pruritus, whatever the cause. In the atopic child with asthma it is worth remembering that episodes of pruritus may be induced by an imminent asthmatic attack as can an exacerbation of eczema[17]. Infestations and insect bites are some of the commonest causes of intensely itchy dermatoses; however, the degree of reaction is in part dependent on the host response to the presence of the mite or foreign substances in the bite. Atopic individuals tend to react more fiercely than non-atopics, but a degree of tolerance to bites can develop with repeated exposure. The term papular urticaria is applied to describe a cutaneous, papulo-vesicular reaction occurring on an urticated base in response to insect bites and said to predominantly affect children. Unfortunately this descriptive term does not distinguish clearly between this and other insect bite reactions. Contrary to popular belief pruritus is a common symptom in psoriasis: this is particularly true for extensive psoriasis in which itching may be severe[18].

Dermatitis herpetiformis (Figure 3.4) may frequently be the cause of unexplained pruritus. Intact vesicles are seldom seen as they are rapidly excoriated; distribution of lesions on the extensor surfaces, sacral region and scalp may help, but neurotic excoriations and papular urticaria can produce almost similar eruptions and distribution. In such circumstances a skin biopsy and immunofluorescent

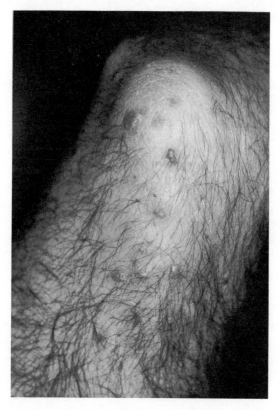

FIGURE 3.4   Dermatitis Herpetiformis: affecting extensor surface of elbow

examination often serves to distinguish. If this is unhelpful a prompt response to a trial course of dapsone may support a diagnosis of dermatitis herpetiformis.

Prolonged pruritus may precede the clinical development of other autoimmune bullous disorders, particularly bullous pemphigoid, and although anti-basement membrane IgG may be present on indirect analysis of sera, this proves specific in less than half the cases[19].

When no apparent dermatosis can be found it is important to ensure that subtle skin changes of scabies, pediculosis, asteatotic eczema and symptomatic dermatographism are not being overlooked.

ITCHING AND SYSTEMIC DISORDERS

The incidence of systemic disease in patients with generalized pruritus, without primary skin disease, has been variously reported as between 10–50%, depending on the criteria used and the patient selection involved[20]. A list of possible causes is given in Table 3.3.

TABLE 3.3 Systemic disorders causing generalized pruritus

Pregnancy, obstructive hepatic and biliary disease
Uraemia and chronic renal failure
Internal malignancy including myeloma, lymphoma and leukaemia
Polycythaemia rubra vera and iron deficiency
Thyroid and neurological diseases
Drug reactions, especially opiates, phenothiazines, and sulphonylureas
Psychogenic

Pregnancy may be associated with itching, for a variety of reasons, in up to 17% of gestations[21]. Pruritus may be directly related to the pregnant state, or a coincidental condition such as scabies, eczema, urticaria, pediculosis or drug eruption. Concentrating on the former group, this can be divided into pruritus gravidarum without primary skin changes and the specific dermatoses of pregnancy which itch.

Pruritus gravidarum usually occurs in the third trimester, and skin changes may occur secondary to scratching; the itching is due to intra-hepatic cholestasis, which may be evident clinically but more often biochemically. In the more severe case of jaundice, pruritus is more likely to have commenced in the first trimester and may progress to a florid cholestasis of pregnancy. The pruritus and jaundice may respond to cholestyramine[21], but in any case will resolve after delivery; it can, however, return in future pregnancies or with oral contraceptive therapy. Itching can occur in virtually all the specific dermatoses of pregnancy: these can be broadly classified as herpes gestationis, a rare bullous pemphigoid-like eruption commencing around the umbilicus, and often preceded by itching, and polymorphic eruption of pregnancy which is common, frequently localized in part to stretch marks, and the rash coincides with the onset of itching (Figure 3.5). This latter type

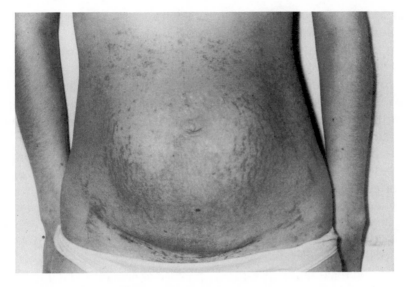

FIGURE 3.5   Polymorphic eruption of pregnancy

corresponds approximately with the American grouping of pruritic papules and plaques of pregnancy, but is a broader classification[22].

Liver disease of various causes, but predominantly cholestatic, is commonly associated with pruritus which often becomes a troublesome symptom. It is frequently presumed to be related to the accumulation of unconjugated bile salts in the skin, but concentrations of bile salts in the skin correspond poorly with the degree of pruritus[23]. Furthermore, although bile salts when applied to abraded skin cause itching, they only achieve this at concentrations in excess of those found in hepatic disease[24]. It therefore seems unlikely that bile salts are the direct cause of itching in such cases. It also remains unclear why certain cholestatic liver disorders such as alcoholic cirrhosis are relatively uncommon causes of pruritus, when itching is almost a constant feature of primary bilary cirrhosis. Interestingly, fulminant hepatic failure may be preceded by a reduction in pruritus, suggesting that a hepatically synthesized pruritogen is aetiologic. Undoubtedly cholestyramine, an ion exchange resin, is partially effective in reducing the itch[25]. The treatment of pruritus in patients with hepatic disease is obviously dependent on its aetiology. It should be remembered that various drugs can cause intrahepatic cholestasis, such as the phenothiazines, tolbutamide and erythromycin estolate; these obviously should be discontinued. However, it is important to remember that not all drug causes of pruritus are via a cholestatic mechanism. If a correctable mechanical obstruction exists this possibility should be explored. Cholestyramine is the mainstay of treatment for cholestatic pruritus, but it can cause problems with malabsorption of fat-soluble vitamins, especially vitamin K; change in bowel habit and hyperchloraemic acidosis can also occur. An alternative is colestipol hydrochloride[3]. Plasma perfusion of charcoal-coated beads has been reported as giving variable relief[23] and ultraviolet light therapy has been documented as successful in a small series of patients with primary biliary cirrhosis[26]. Conventional H_1 antihistamines tend to be ineffective in this situation, but surprisingly terfenadine has been reported as helpful[27].

Chronic renal failure is a common cause of generalized itching, but unfortunately haemodialysis can precipitate the problem as well as improve it. Young et al[28] found that up to 85% of patients on haemodialysis suffered with pruritus. A third of these were itching before dialysis and the rest after; 12% noticed a reduction in itching after six months dialysis. They proposed that there was one definite and two possible positive correlations: a firm association with the pre-dialysis blood urea, and tentative correlations with the degree of asteatosis and secondary hyperparathyroidism. In the case of the latter, relief was obtained by subtotal parathyroidectomy, but later recurred. Certainly, dry skin does seem to be an aggravating problem in chronic renal failure especially those on high dose diuretic regimens (Figure 3.6).

The reason for itching in uraemia remains obscure. Obviously, urea is not the direct cause otherwise dialysis would be more beneficial; because pruritus is uncommon in acute renal failure it would seem likely that one, or several, slowly accumulated pruritogens are responsible. Lowering the dialysate magnesium concentration has been described as beneficial[29]; however, the mainstay of therapy at present is the use of ultraviolet B phototherapy. Blachley et al[30] noticed that the improvement of pruritus following UVB therapy was associated with a reduction of skin phosphorus to normal values and proposed that itching may be the result of microprecipitation of calcium and

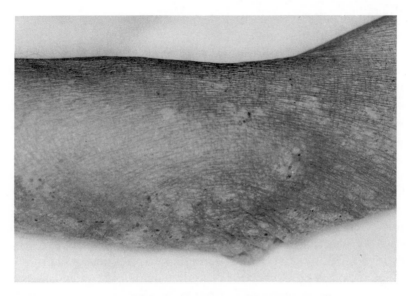

FIGURE 3.6   Dry skin and lichenification in chronic renal failure: changes on arm shown

magnesium phosphate in the skin. Numerous other treatments have been tried to relieve the problem, two of which are worthy of consideration, the use of oral cholestyramine[31], and activated charcoal[32]. A cautionary tale of scabies masquerading as uraemic pruritus in a dialysis unit[33] reminds one that common causes of itching may occur in any situation.

Haematological disorders and lymphomas can cause generalized pruritus. Iron-deficient anaemia has been linked to itching, and an improvement with replacement therapy observed[34], but iatrogenic iron deficiency,by therapeutic venesection, failed to precipitate pruritus in another study[35], perhaps suggesting an intermediate mechanism. Male patients with unexplained iron deficiency and pruritus have a high incidence of internal malignancy[34].

Pruritus is a recognized complication of polycythaemia rubra vera. The trigger factor appears to be sudden cooling of the skin, such as encountered after bathing; platelets may be involved in the release of pruritogens, such as prostaglandin E_2 and serotonin. The irritation is at least partially responsive to aspirin[14]; cimetidine, pizotifen and cyproheptadine may be alternatives[3].

Severe generalized pruritus is a major clinical problem in Hodgkin's disease and may denote a poorer prognosis[36]. The mechanism is poorly understood, but it may respond to cimetidine or alternatively improve as chemotherapy induces control[37]. Both mycosis fungoides and Sézary syndrome can also cause pruritus; recently a case of the latter has been reported to respond favourably to cyclosporin-A, both in terms of reduction in itching and of tumour mass[38]. Myelomatosis[39] and leukaemia may also occasionally present with generalized pruritus (Figure 3.7).

Internal carcinoma is a rare but important cause of itching. It is most often seen in lung, breast, colonic and gastric tumours, but this probably just reflects the incidence of these neoplasms and it may occur in virtually any visceral carcinoma. Infrequently pruritus and malignancy may be associated in acquired ichthyosis, and this is usually with small bowel lymphomas, but may also be seen with visceral carcinomas (Figure 3.8).

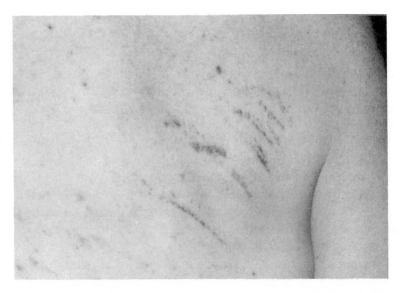

FIGURE 3.7 Haemorrhagic scratch marks in acute myeloid leukaemia: changes shown over back

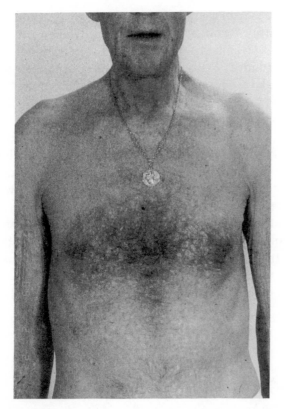

FIGURE 3.8   Dry skin and pruritus: occurring in a patient with underlying bronchial carcinoma

Brain tumours are a rare cause of itching; this can either be localized to the nostril, in the case of a tumour invading the base of the fourth ventricle, or generalized[40]. In the case of the latter and with many malignancies the mechanism is obscure. Other neurological factors have been documented as causing pruritus, such as strokes[41], brain abscesses[42] and multiple sclerosis[43]. The symptoms are frequently unilateral or of an unusual distribution and may be paroxysmal. These rare occurrences help confirm the role of cortical function in itch appreciation.

Endocrine disorders can be associated with itching, but this is less common than traditionally taught. Hyperthyroidism is infrequently a cause, the mechanism is again obscure; in hypothyroidism the association is probably secondary to asteatosis. Diabetes has often been incriminated as an endocrinological cause of itching, but this is almost certainly unfounded. Pruritus in diabetes is usually crural and secondary to candida; perhaps tolbutamide-induced cholestasis, or other therapy-linked causes of pruritus are also responsible for diabetes' undeserved reputation.

Senile and idiopathic pruritus should be diagnosed by exclusion. Unfortunately the degree of itching may be severe, and although non-specific measures such as $\frac{1}{2}\%$ menthol or phenol in aqueous cream, emollient preparations and sedative antihistamines are worth trying; in severe cases they are of only partial value. Where there is associated depression, doxepin hydrochloride, a tricyclic antidepressant with H_1 antihistamine properties may be helpful. A recent double-blind placebo-controlled trial of oxatomide in pruritus senilis has suggested it may be of value[44]. Systemic steroids are occasionally used in extreme cases, but the short-term benefits are seldom worth the long-term hazards.

LOCALIZED ITCHING

This is more likely to be due to primary skin disease than in the case of generalized pruritus. However, there are some important systemic causes that should not be forgotten, e.g. the previously mentioned rare cause of nasal itching secondary to a brain tumour. Other examples are Paget's disease (particularly extramammary Paget's effecting the ano-genital region and associated with internal adenocarcinoma), invasive squamous carcinoma with multifocal pigmented Bowen's disease[45] and Crohn's disease also principally affecting the perineal area. Parasitic infections may give rise to localized pruritus, and this can vary from the common threadworm infection, predominantly in children, causing pruritus ani, to the rarer Far-Eastern acquired Gnathostomiasis infestation which often presents cutaneously with localized erythema, itching or pain, at virtually any site on the body[46]. It is interesting to note that the yeasts in the perianal region are often saprophytic, whereas dermatophytes are likely to be pathogenic[47]. Infectious vaginitis and trichomoniasis are, however, common causes of localized vulval irritation, especially in diabetics. They are usually associated with a vaginal discharge, which is often a helpful clue.

There are several areas on the body that seem to be particularly prone to develop self-perpetuating forms of itching, e.g. lichen simplex chronicus. In this, a presumed previous prolonged stimulus, such as eczema, is thought to have caused post-inflammatory cutaneous hyperalgesia, in which spontaneous triggering of itch receptors occurs, despite loss of the original stimulus. The cutaneous changes of lichenification and thickening develop in response to the subsequent scratching; the nape of neck, anterior shin, extensor surface of forearm and ano-genital areas are particularly prone. There often seems to be underlying emotional factors that exacerbate this problem. Occasionally there is overlap with papular and nodular prurigo, and these tend to be rather more extensive and produce severe scratching problems in which multiple discrete nodules occur, in association with histologically demonstrable cutaneous nerve hypertrophy.

Many skin diseases may, at some time in their genesis, be local causes of irritation. There are, however, some specific causes of itching, such as Fox–Fordyce disease (Figure 3.9), a form of apocrine miliaria affecting mainly the axillae, but these are comparatively rare. Some of the dermatoses that commonly, but not exclusively, affect the ano-genital region are given in Table 3.4. Pruritus ani is a common problem, which is difficult to clear permanently. It may be related to primary skin disease, be caused by systemic disease, some of which have previously been mentioned, or be idiopathic, in which constitutional and psychological influences may be especially important. Pruritus ani is more common in males than females: in the latter it is often associated with pruritus vulvae. Males, however, are more likely to have a definite cause than females[48]. Probably the commonest cause of pruritus ani is an irritant reaction to a combination of minor faecal contamination and moisture acting as skin irritants in an area which is often hot, occluded by tight clothing and well-supplied with neurovascular inputs. Consequently, this area appears to have a lower threshold for itching to occur and despite attracting social embarrassment is often found to be a particularly pleasurable area to scratch! Careful attention to anal hygiene, with gentle, post-defaecation cleansing of the perianal area with water and cotton wool, or mild astringents

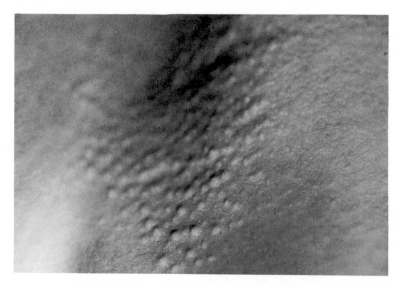

FIGURE 3.9   Fox–Fordyce disease: affecting the axilla

TABLE 3.4 Causes of localized ano-genital irritation

Endogenous eczemas especially seborrhoeic eczema and intertrigo
Exogenous allergic and particularly irritant contact eczemas
Infections with dermatophytes, candida and trichomonas
Lichen simplex, lichen planus and lichen sclerosus et atrophicus
Psoriasis and some autoimmune bullous disorders
Malignancy and dysplasias
Haemorrhoids, skin tags and fissures
Psychogenic causes

such as $\frac{1}{4}$% aqueous silver nitrate lotion, is probably the most important aspect of management[49]. A change to looser garments is an obvious aid in all forms of ano-genital pruritus. The use of 1% hydrocortisome cream and/or a nocturnal dose of sedative antihistamine may help initially.

Many of the factors involved with perianal irritation are common to genital itching. Pruritus vulvae is frequently encountered, scrotal pruritus also occurs, but perhaps less commonly seeking referral.

In ano-genital pruritus topical polypharmacy by the patient, with proprietary topical anaesthetic and germicidal preparations, is commonplace. Taking cosmetics, deodorants and clothing chemicals into account, together with prescribed topical therapies, it is not surprising that allergic and irritant contact eczema to these substances is a frequent occurrence. For example, a common medically-approved lubricant, KY jelly, contains parabens, which can occasionally act as a contact allergen. Both perianal and genital skin absorb topical steroids very effectively, so if necessary, weak, or preferably bland, preparations should be used. Potent topical steroids applied for more than a short period will result in thinning of the skin, which may exacerbate cutaneous hyperalgesia and so increase itching, particularly in atrophic vaginitis, a common post-menopausal cause of pruritus vulvae. A difficult problem is encountered in lichen sclerosus et atrophicus, where the inflammatory component is helped, but the subsequent skin fragility is enhanced by topical steroids.

As with other forms of pruritus, the most important aspect of management is accurate assessment of its cause, but in localized anal and genital itching especially, the patient may be acutely embarrassed as well as tormented by the problem and deserves a sympathetic and attentive approach.

References

1. Neville, R. G. (1985). Pruritus: a 'coat of many colours'. *J. R. Coll. Gen. Pract.,* **35,** 23–8
2. Mikuni, I. (1984). Eye itching in ophthalmology and its treatment. *Tokai J. Exp. Clin. Med.,* **9,** 415–9
3. Denman, S. T. (1986). A review of pruritus. *J. Am. Acad. Dermatol.,* **14,** 375–92
4. Bowden, K., Brown, B. G. and Batty, J. E. (1954). 5 hydroxytryptamine: Its occurrence in cowhage. *Nature,* **174,** 925–6
5. Tuckett, R. P. (1982). Itch evoked by electrical stimulation of the skin. *J. Invest. Dermatol.,* **79,** 368–73
6. Martin, J. (1985). Pruritus. *Int. J. Dermatol.,* **24,** 634–9
7. Bickford, R. G. (1938). Experiments relating to the itch sensation, its peripheral mechanism and central pathways. *Clin. Sci.,* **3,** 377–86
8. Scott, P. V. and Fischer, H. B. J. (1982). Spinal opiate analgesia and facial pruritus: a neural theory. *Postgrad. Med. J.,* **58,** 531–5
9. Taubman, S. M. and Spielman, M. (1979). Tungiasis: A case report. *J. Am. Podiatr. Med. Assoc.,* **69,** 383–4

10. Ferguson, M. M., Simpson, N. B. and Hammersley, N. (1984). The treatment of erosive lichen planus with a retinoid-etretinate. *Oral Medicine, 58*, 283–7
11. Brenner, S., Ophir, J. and Krakowski, A. (1984). Pediculid: An unusual -id reaction to pediculosis capitis. *Dermatologica, 168*, 189–91
12. Champion, R. H. (1984). Generalised pruritus. *Br. Med. J., 289*, 751–3
13. Arnold, H. L. (1984). Paroxysmal pruritus: Its clinical characterisation and hypothesis of its pathogenesis. *J. Am. Acad. Dermatol., 11*, 322–6
14. Kligman, A. M., Greaves, M. W. and Steinman, H. (1986). Water-induced itching without cutaneous signs. *Arch. Dermatol., 122*, 183–6
15. Fjellner, B. and Hagermark, O. (1979). Pruritus in polycythaemia vera: Treatment with aspirin and possibility of platelet involvement. *Acta. Dermatol. Venereol. (Stockh.), 59*, 505–12
16. Greenwood, R. and Barker, D. J. (1985). Pruritus and atopy in Asians. *Clin. Exp. Dermatol., 10*, 179–81
17. David, T. J., Wybrew, M. and Hennessen, U. (1984). Prodromal itching in childhood asthma. *Lancet, 2*, 154–5
18. Gratton, C. E. H. (1985). Itch in Psoriasis. *Bristol Med. Chir. J., 100*, 36/42
19. Bingham, E. A., Burrows, D. and Sandord, J. C. (1984). Prolonged pruritus and bullous pemphigoid. *Clin. Exp. Dermatol., 9*, 564–70
20. Jorizzo, J. L. (1983). The itchy patient: A practical approach. *Primary Care, 10*, 339–53
21. Winton, G. B. and Lewis, C. W. (1982). Dermatoses of pregnancy. *J. Am. Acad. Dermatol., 6*, 977–98
22. Holmes, R. C. and Black, M. M. (1982). The specific dermatoses of pregnancy: A reappraisal with special emphasis on a proposed simplified classification. *Clin. Exp. Dermatol., 7*, 65–73
23. Greaves, M. W. (1982). The nature and management of pruritus. *Practitioner, 226*, 1223–5
24. Ghent, C. N. and Bloomer, J. R. (1979). Itch in liver disease: Facts and speculations. *Yale J. Biol. Med., 52*, 77–82
25. Carey, J. B. and Williams, G. (1961). Relief of pruritus of jaundice with a bile-acid sequestering resin. *J. Am. Med. Assoc., 176*, 432–5
26. Perlstein, S. M. (1981). Phototherapy for primary biliary cirrhosis. *Arch. Dermatol., 117*, 608–11
27. Duncan, J. S., Kennedy, H. J. and Triger, D. R. (1984). Treatment of pruritus due to chronic obstructive liver disease. *Br. Med. J., 289*, 22
28. Young, A. W., Sweeney, E. W., David, D. S., Cheigh, J., Hochgelerent, E. L., Sakai, S., Stenzel, K. H. and Rubin, A. L. (1973). Dermatologic evaluation of pruritus in patients on hemodialysis. *N. Y. State J. Med., 73*, 2670–4
29. Graf, H., Kovarik, J., Stummvoll, H. K. and Wolf, S. (1979). Disappearance of uraemic pruritus after lowering dialysate magnesium concentration. *Br. Med. J., 2*, 1478–9
30. Blachley, J. D., Blankenship, D. M., Menter, A., Parker, T. F. and Knochel, J. P. (1985). Uremic pruritus skin divalent ion content and response to ultra violet phototherapy. *Am. J. Kidney Dis., 5*, 237–41
31. Silverberg, D. S., Iaina, A., Reisin, E., Rotzak, R. and Eliahou, H. E. (1977). Cholestyramine in uraemic pruritus. *Br. Med. J., 1*, 752–3
32. Pederson, J. A., Matter, B. J., Czerwinski, A. W. and Llach, F. (1980). Relief of idiopathic generalised pruritus in dialysis patients with activated oral charcoal.

Ann. Int. Med., **93,** 446–8

33. Lempert, K. D., Baltz, P. S., Welton, W. A. and Whittier, F. C. (1985). Pseudo-uremic pruritus: A scabies epidemic in a dialysis unit. *Am. J. Kidney Dis.,* **5,** 117–19

34. Vickers, C. F. H. (1974). Nutrition and skin: Iron deficiency. In Ledingham, J. C. G. *Proceedings of the Tenth Symposium on Advanced Medicine,* pp. 311–16. (London: Pitmans)

35. Tucker, W. F. G., Briggs, C. and Challoner, T. (1984). Absence of pruritus in iron deficiency following venesection. *Clin. Exp. Dermatol.,* **9,** 186–9

36. Feiner, A. S., Mahmood, T. and Wallner, S. F. (1978). Prognostic importance of pruritus in Hodgkin's disease. *J. Am. Med. Assoc.,* **240,** 2738–40

37. Aymard, J. P., Lederlin, P., Witz, F., Colomb. J. N., Herbeuval, R. and Webber, B. (1980). Cimetidine for pruritus in Hodgkin's disease. *Br. Med. J.,* **280,** 151–2

38. Totterman, T. H., Scheynius, A., Killander, A., Danersund, A. and Alm, G. V. (1985). Treatment of therapy-resistant Sezary Syndrome with cyclosporin-A: Suppression of pruritus, leukaemic T cell activation markers and tumour mass. *Scand. J. Haematol.,* **34,** 196–203

39. Erskine, J. G., Rowan, R. M., Alexander, J. O'D. and Sekoni, G. A. (1977). ritus as a presentation of myelomatosis. *Br. Med. J.,* **1,** 687–8

40. Andreev, V. C. and Petkov, I. (1975). Skin manifestations associated with tumours of the brain. *Br. J. Dermatol.,* **92,** 675–8

41. Massey, E. W. (1984). Unilateral neurogenic pruritus following a stroke. *Stroke,* **15,** 901–3

42. Sullivan, M. J. and Drake, M. E. (1984). Unilateral pruritus and nocardia brain abscess. *Neurology,* **34,** 828–9

43. Osterman, P. O. and Westerberg, C. E. (1975). Paroxysmal attacks in multiple sclerosis. *Brain,* **98,** 189–202

44. Dupont, C., de Maubeuge, J., Kotlar, W., Lays, Y and Masson, M. (1984). Oxatomide in the treatment of pruritus senilis. A double-blind placebo-controlled trial. *Dermatologica,* **169,** 348–53

45. Powell, F. C. and Perry, H. O. (1985). Pruritus ani: Could it be malignant? *Geriatrics,* **40,** 89–91

46. Kagen, C. N., Vance, J. C. and Simpson, M. (1984). Gnathostomiasis: Infestation in an Asian immigrant. *Arch. Dermatol.,* **120,** 508–10

47. Dodi, G., Pirone, E., Bettin, A., Veller, C., Infantino, A., Pianon, P., Mortellaro, L. M. and Lise, M. (1985). The mycotic flora in proctological patients with or without pruritus ani. *Br. J. Surg.,* **72,** 967–9

48. Verbov, J. (1984). Pruritus ani and its management: Study and reappraisal. *Clin. Exp. Dermatol.,* **9,** 46–52

49. Alexander-Williams, J. (1983). Causes and management of anal irritation. *Br. Med. J.,* **287,** 1528

4

TRACE ELEMENTS

M. M. MOLOKHIA

INTRODUCTION

An element can be classified as either a bulk or trace element according to its concentration in plant or animal tissue. In man, the borderline may be drawn at 100 ppm. Chemical analysis shows a striking similarity between the chemical composition of living matter and that of the Earth's crust. Unlike other organs, the skin is in direct contact with the environment with its wide array of irritants, sensitizers, toxins and generally reactive constituents.

Metals and their compounds have been present in man's environment since the dawn of history and were utilized at a very early stage in skin therapy. The ability to understand the biological significance of trace elements was hampered for a long time by the lack of accurate analytical techniques. The discovery of the essential role of iron more than two centuries ago was largely enhanced by the presence of this metal in bulk concentrations in peripheral blood. More elements have since been discovered to have an essential role, although the majority of trace elements are still considered nonessential. With modern technology in chemical analysis and easy accessibility of the skin it should be possible to advance our understanding of these microconstituents. The numerous enzyme activities exhibited by the skin are a reflection of the metabolic role of that organ. These enzymes depend in turn on the presence of specific metal ions. The unique processes of keratinization and melanin formation are enzyme-dependent and therefore could be influenced by trace metal deficiencies or excesses. Even

TABLE 4.1   Trace element concentration in abdominal skin

Element	No. of samples	Epidermis (μg/g dry weight)[a]	Dermis (μg/g dry weight)[a]
Zn	36	70.5 ± 26.3	12.6 ± 4.7
Cu	23	7.01 ± 2.36	3.13 ± 0.99
Mn	34	1.98 ± 0.37	0.27 ± 0.13
Fe	16	82.4 ± 33.8	24.6 ± 12.0
Rb	24	6.62 ± 2.32	3.47 ± 1.43
Se	36	0.52 ± 0.14	0.39 ± 0.09
Au	14	0.0087 ± 0.0061	0.0019 ± 0.0016
Sb	10	0.133 ± 0.028	0.028 ± 0.019

[a] Values are expressed as mean ± S.D.

essential trace elements like iron can become toxic if excessive accumulation takes place, as in haemochromatosis. It is hard to imagine that idiopathic overload states exist only in relation to iron, and possibly copper, among all the elements in the periodic table.

TRACE ELEMENT CONCENTRATION IN SKIN

The skin does not rank high among body organs for its trace element content. There appear to be little differences between the sexes, races or different age groups with regard to elemental composition of the skin. However, regional anatomical variations exist which makes comparison of values obtained from different sites rather difficult[1]. Table 4.1 shows the concentration of some essential and non-essential trace elements in abdominal skin as found by neutron activation analysis in the Manchester area. Both groups of elements were found in significantly higher concentrations in epidermis relative to dermis. This may suggest an excretory role for the epidermis with regard to trace elements. However, the higher epidermal content of essential elements like zinc and copper may reflect its enzymic metabolic activity.

PERCUTANEOUS ABSORPTION OF METALS

The skin is impermeable to most metals in the non-ionic state. However, in ionic form many metal compounds penetrate the skin barrier very easily[2,3]. The rate of penetration will depend on valency state and the vehicle used. Metal objects coming in contact with the skin may also be dissolved by the chemical action of sweat and subsequently absorbed; examples are copper[4] and nickel[5]. Absorption of metallic compounds through unbroken skin is responsible for the allergic reactions to nickel, chromium, cobalt and mercury in sensitized individuals. The bulk of cutaneous absorption takes place across the horny cell layer. A significant proportion is channelled through hair follicles and sweat ducts. This makes certain anatomical sites such as the axilla more susceptible to metal absorption. Foreign body granuloma developing in axillary skin from the use of deodorant lotions containing zirconium salts, is an example.

METAL ACCUMULATION, BINDING AND ELIMINATION BY THE SKIN

Under normal conditions, essential trace metals do not accumulate in the skin or in its appendages. Analytical data have shown very high concentrations of some metals in melanosomes, but the role they may play in this highly specialized organelle remains completely unknown[6]. Following therapeutic use, some metals are deposited in the skin where they are slowly eliminated. This happens when gold is given intramuscularly in rheumatoid arthritis. The concentration of gold was measured in skin biopsies from seven patients who received sodium aurothiomalate injections (Table 4.2). The results show that very high levels of gold were detectable more than two years after cessation of therapy.

Other heavy metals like silver and mercury may accumulate in the skin from topical use. They bind strongly with proteins in general and with those containing abundant sulphydryl groups in particular. Occupational argyria has long been known in silver workers although such cases are becoming less common with a better working environment. Bleehen and his co-workers[7] reported this condition in five

TABLE 4.2 Gold levels in abdominal skin following therapy in rheumatoid arthritis patients

Case No.	Weeks since therapy	Epidermis (μg/g dry weight)	Dermis (μg/g dry weight)
1	1	80.80	22.00
2	1	29.80	40.40
3	2	24.60	9.94
4	2	4.27	26.60
5	4	8.42	20.50
6	16	1.18	0.58
7	130	0.07	0.28
Control skin		0.0087 ($\pm$0.0061)	0.0019 ($\pm$0.0016)

furnace-men employed in extracting silver from its ores in Sheffield. Using X-ray microanalysis, they demonstrated silver-containing granules in dermal macrophages, elastic and collagen fibrils as well as in the basal lamina of epidermis, sweat glands and blood vessels. They also showed the presence of mercury, titanium and selenium in the same ultrastructural localization. Although no identifiable silver-containing granules were found in the epidermis itself, this did not seem to rule out the presence of excessive amounts of silver in a more soluble form.

Natural desquamation of the skin plays only a small part in the excretion of both essential and nonessential trace elements[8]. An increase in skin desquamation is sometimes seen after exposure to heavy metals and hair and nails may also be shed as a result of this toxic effect. Thallium acetate used to be given to children with scalp ringworm to cause epilation, as part of the treatment, before griseofulvin was discovered. Complete elimination of a toxic element from the body may still be followed by complications years later. Arsenic is a clear example where neoplastic changes may appear in the skin 30 years or longer after its use.

METALS AND SKIN SENSITIZATION

The capacity of metals to cause sensitization of the skin varies considerably. Metal dermatitis is most frequently caused by nickel, chromates and mercury. Dissolution of metals like nickel into sweat is believed to be a first stage in the allergic reaction. Using an artificial sweat formulation, Hemingway and Molokhia[5] found that the rate of dissolution of nickel was dependent on the acidity of the solution, temperature and the presence of oxygen in the system. They suggested that allergic reactions to nickel may be minimized by using a barrier cream containing a reducing agent.

Upon entry into skin, metal ions combine with proteins to form antigens. Such antigens lead to a cell-mediated type of delayed hypersensitivity in susceptible individuals. Although reactions may follow oral challenge with metallic salts, there is no proof that dietary intake is responsible for exacerbations of metal dermatitis. In a double-blind cross-over study of 24 women and two men with proven nickel dermatitis, Gawkrodger and co-workers[9] showed that pompholyx could only be induced by oral challenge with nickel in excess of 5 mg. This was far in excess of the normal daily intake from a typical Western-style diet (less than 0.5 mg) and therefore it seemed unlikely that systemically absorbed nickel played a significant role in such eruptions.

TRACE ELEMENT DEFICIENCIES AND SKIN DISEASE

Because of the ubiquitous presence of trace elements in most diets and the growing dependence of man on imported food, deficiency states are rarely caused by deficient intake. Increased loss from the body or increased demand by tissues are more frequently relevant in manifest deficiency. Trace elements could also be chelated by dietary constituents such as phytates or by chelating drugs like penicillamine.

Changes in skin or its appendages due to trace element deficiencies are usually nonspecific and may mimic well-known disorders. The association between iron deficiency anaemia and koilonychia is well-known although normal infants under one year of age frequently have flattened nails. Severe pruritus is a well-known manifestation of iron deficiency anaemia and it can be promptly relieved by iron supplements[10].

Menkes kinky hair syndrome is a genetically determined disease (sex-linked recessive) caused by defective copper absorption. The abnormal hair keratinization in this disease gives it a characteristic steel wire appearance. Microscopic examination of hair invariably shows a twisted pattern (pili torti) in both patients and carriers.

Deficiency of cobalt in its biochemically active form (vitamin B12) has been found to cause generalized hyperpigmentation of the skin, particularly over the small joints of the hands and feet[11]. Other pigmentary changes involving hair and nails described in association with pernicious anaemia were completely reversible by treatment with cyanocobalamin[12].

Zinc deficiency has a marked effect on the skin and hair in most animal species including man. Deficient animals develop a skin eruption which resembles psoriasis both clinically and histologically. This association has stimulated interest in studying the role of zinc in the body in general. However, the enthusiasm in investigating zinc status in psoriasis shown in the early 1970s has been dampened by discouraging results from therapeutic trials with zinc in this very common disease. Recent studies have confirmed that serum zinc levels are not lowered in psoriasis except perhaps in the extensive pustular form[13].

Zinc deficiency states in man may result from inadequate parenteral feeding or the administration of drugs like penicillamine[14] or anticonvulsants[15]. The full syndrome of zinc deficiency is seen in the rare inherited disease acrodermatitis enteropathica (AE). It is nearly 15 years since zinc was first used to treat both AE and AE-like syndromes. Although most workers agree that serum zinc levels are low in these conditions, there has been no convincing evidence to show that tissue zinc is also lowered. The response of such patients to zinc supplements, in spite of normal tissue levels, seems to be a paradox and the mechanism of improvement with zinc treatment remains unknown.

The skin lesions in AE are not specific and may consist of scaly erythema and pustules with erosions around body orifices. Hair and nails are also affected and total alopecia may develop. It is not clear whether these inflammatory skin lesions are due to neutrophilic activation, an associated cutaneous infection, a defect in neutrophil activity or some other metabolic or immunological abnormality. The effects of zinc on the host immune response were reviewed in a recent article[16]. It seems that this element influences most aspects of such response beginning with the generation of specific recognizing proteins and ending with the production of specific and nonspecific effectors of inflammation.

THERAPEUTIC USES OF ELEMENTS

Metals and their compounds have been used since ancient times for their therapeutic as well as cosmetic effects on skin. Non-metallic elements like iodine and sulphur figure prominently in world pharmacopoeias as useful topical agents. Heavy elements like lead, bismuth and thallium have been largely abandoned because of their toxic effects. Arsenic used to occupy a very special place in skin therapy. Its uses covered a wide range of skin diseases as well as general disorders and infections. However, it has virtually ceased to be used in man being superseded by more effective and less toxic drugs. Skin neoplasms and keratoses are still occasionally seen in elderly patients with a history of arsenical ingestion during earlier years.

The following account describes elements in current use and their applications.

Aluminium

Alum, which is the mixed sulphate of aluminium and potassium, has been used since the middle ages for its astringent action on skin and also to treat hyperhidrosis. Modern preparations contain aluminium chloride hexahydrate, which is a more potent inhibitor of sweat, as a 20% solution in an alcoholic base. Aluminium acetate solution is used as a skin disinfectant and cleansing agent. Powdered aluminium oxide in different particle size grades is used in 40–60% paste as an abrasive agent for the treatment of acne.

Antimony

Antimony was used by the ancients as both a medicine and a cosmetic. Its use was revived early this century when organic antimony compounds were introduced as parasiticides. In dermatology, antimonials are used intramuscularly for the treatment of leishmaniasis.

Copper

Copper sulphate is still used in some countries as a mild astringent and antiseptic preparation. It has been used in the past with limited success to treat the skin in vitiligo[17]. Copper acetate has been added in a very low concentration to a keratolytic wart removal formula, although the manufacturers have not stated what specific action it might have. Traces of copper have been shown to be dissolved by sweat and absorbed through the skin from bracelets worn by arthritic patients[18].

Gold

Gold therapy was used at the beginning of this century in the treatment of lupus erythematosus. This disease was erroneously believed to be a manifestation of tuberculosis and was therefore treated with the same agents available. There has been renewed interest in gold therapy for chronic discoid L.E[19].

Iodine

Tincture of iodine, which usually causes considerable pain when applied to wounds, has largely been replaced by newer water-soluble iodine compounds. Povidone-iodine is used as a spray, bath concentrate or a scalp application for the treatment of seborrhoeic dermatitis and superficial infections. Oral treatment with potassium iodide is used in deep fungal infections like sporotrichosis.

Mercury

The use of mercuric chloride as an antiseptic lotion has declined in recent years. However, mercury compounds are still available as creams or ointments and sold over the counter in many parts of the world for their bleaching effects on dark skin. Although they inhibit melanin production, their prolonged use may lead to greyish discoloration due to deposition of the metal.

Selenium

Selenium disulphide was found to have an antimitotic effect on the epidermis. It is commonly used as a shampoo in a concentration of 2.5% to treat seborrhoeic dermatitis of the scalp. Manufacturers recommend that selenium-containing shampoos should not be used more than twice weekly and that their use should be discontinued after initial control. The same preparation is sometimes used in the treatment of pityriasis versicolor.

Silicon

Silicones are inert organic compounds of silicon. Because of their versatile properties they have found many applications in industry and medicine. They impart a barrier effect on the skin and offer protection against irritation. They also act as water repellents and prevent maceration caused by wet skin conditions. Creams and gels containing dimethicone are widely used in napkin dermatitis, pressure sores and in stoma care.

Silver

Silver nitrate is a mild astringent when used in weak aqueous solution and can be very useful in treating exudative skin conditions. It is also used on a short-term basis in the treatment of leg ulcers to stop excessive granulation. Sticks covered with toughened silver nitrate and alum are used for cauterizing aphthous ulcers and minor skin lesions.

Sulphur

The parasiticidal action of elemental sulphur has long been recognized. Sulphur ointment (BP) was the standard treatment for scabies until the Second World War. Sulphur also has a mild keratolytic effect which is helpful in acne and dandruff. Sixteen acne preparations currently listed in the BNF Number 12 (1986) contain sulphur in a concentration of 2–10%. Sulphur (0.5–2.0%) in aqueous cream is thought to be effective as a topical application in rosacea.

Titanium

Titanium is the tenth most abundant element in the Earth's crust. Its compounds are used mainly on the skin as protective agents. The oxide is an inert substance used in pastes and ointments for the treatment of napkin dermatitis and bed sores. The bright white colour of the powder makes it ideal for use as an opaque reflectant in sunscreens.

Zinc

Zinc compounds are probably the most widely used preparations of any metal on the skin. Their use goes back in history to Ancient Egypt when calamine (zinc carbonate) was mined from ores containing traces of ferric oxide. The presence of this reddish pigment gave the product cosmetic acceptability. Today, it is added deliberately to the purified substance. Calamine in the form of lotion or cream has a soothing and cooling effect on the skin and is used mainly in pruritic conditions.

Insoluble zinc oxide is widely incorporated in dusting powders, pastes, ointments and creams as an inert vehicle. However, soluble zinc impurities can easily be detected in the oxide and could therefore be absorbed from these formulations[20]. Zinc pyrithione is an effective antidandruff agent and is widely available in shampoo form. Zinc sulphate as 1% lotion was used in treating leg ulcers long before the role of zinc in wound healing was discovered. Zinc chloride is sometimes used as a 30–40% paste to eradicate superficial malignant skin lesions in what has become known as Mohs surgery[21].

Oral zinc therapy has now been in use for more than two decades. It was first used to treat zinc-deficient dwarfs in the Middle East[22]. It proved to be life-saving in acrodermatitis enteropathica[23] and has since been used in acne[24], alopecia areata[25] and dissecting cellulitis of the scalp[26]. Long-term therapy with oral zinc was also found to restore eyebrow hair growth in leprosy patients[27]. Other salts of zinc have been used orally and these are currently available as capsules, effervescent tablets and syrup. The therapeutic dose of zinc sulphate of 200 mg 1–3 times daily was modelled on that of ferrous sulphate given in iron deficiency anaemia. This is not based on any experimental basis and seems to be much higher than daily requirements.

Zirconium

Zirconium salts are used to control axillary hyperhidrosis. Like all other metallic ions, Zr^{2+} is a protein precipitant and a strong binder to keratin. This results in closure of sweat pores and asymptomatic retention of sweat. The use of zirconium lactate in antiperspirants and deodorants has been largely replaced by zirconyl oxychloride, because of the former's association with allergic skin granulomas[28].

References

1. Molokhia, M. M. and Portnoy, B. (1970). Neutron activation analysis of trace elements in skin. IV. Regional variations in copper, manganese and zinc in normal skin. *Br. J. Dermatol.,* **82,** 254–5
2. Lloyd, G. K. (1980) Dermal absorption and conjugation of nickel in relation to the induction of allergic contact dermatitis. In Brown, S. S. and Sunderman, F. W. (eds), *Nickel Toxicology,* p. 145. (New York: Academic Press)
3. Bork, K., Morsches, B. and Holzmann, H. (1973) Mercury absorption out of ammoniated mercury ointment. *Arch. Dermatol. Forsch.,* **248,** 137–43
4. Taylor, A. (1985) Therapeutic uses of trace elements. *Clin. Endocrinol. Metab.,* **14,** 703–24

5. Hemingway, J. D. and Molokhia, M. M. (1987) The dissolution of metallic nickel in artificial sweat. *Contact Dermatitis,* **16,** 99–105
6. Seiji, M., Fitzpatrick, T. B., Simpson, R. T. and Birbeck, M. S. (1963) Chemical composition and terminology of specialized organelles (Melanosomes and melanin granules) in mammalian melanocytes. *Nature (London),* **197,** 1082–4
7. Bleehen, S. S., Gould, D. J., Harrington, C. I., Durrant, T. E., Slater, D. M. and Underwood, J. C. E. (1981) Occupational argyria; light and electron microscopic studies and x-ray microanalysis. *Br. J. Dermatol.,* **104,** 19–26
8. Molin, L. and Wester, P. O. (1976) The estimated daily loss of trace elements from normal skin by desquamation. *Scand. J. Clin. Lab. Invest.,* **36,** 679–82
9. Gawkrodger, D. J., Cook, S. W., Fell, G. S. and Hunter, J. A. A. (1986) Nickel dermatitis: the reaction to oral nickel challenge. *Br. J. Dermatol.,* **115,** 33–8
10. Vickers, C. F. H. (1977) Iron deficiency pruritus. *J. Am. Med. Assoc.,* **238,** 129
11. Baker, S. J., Ignatius, M. B., Johnson, S. and Vaish S. K. (1963) Hyper-pigmentation of the skin: a sign of vitamin B12 deficiency. *Br. Med. J.,* **1,** 1713–15
12. Carmel, R. (1985) Hair and finger nail changes in acquired and congenital pernicious anaemia. *Arch. Intern. Med.,* **145,** 484–5
13. Dreno, B., Vandermeeren, M. A., Boiteau, H. L., Stalder, J. F. and Barriere, H. (1986) Plasma zinc is decreased only in generalised pustular psoriasis. *Dermatologica,* **173,** 209–12
14. Klingberg, W. G., Prasad, A. S. and Oberleas, D. (1976) Zinc deficiency following penicillamine therapy. In Prasad, A. S. (ed) *Trace Elements in Human Health and Disease* Vol I, p. 51. (New York: Academic Press)
15. Lewis-Jones, M. S., Evans, S. and Culshaw, M. A. (1985) Cutaneous manifestations of zinc deficiency during treatment with anticonvulsants. *Br. Med. J.,* **290,** 603–4
16. Norris, D. (1985) Zinc and cutaneous inflammation. *Arch. Dermatol.,* **121,** 985–9
17. El-Mofty, A. M. (1957) New clinical findings in the treatment of leucoderma (the effect of the addition of copper to psoralen treatment). *Acta Dermatovenereologica,* Proceedings of the Eleventh International Congress of Dermatology, *Stockholm,* **2,** 539–50
18. Walker, W. R. and Keats, D. M. (1976) Investigations of therapeutic value of copper bracelet in dermal assimilation of copper in arthritic rheumatoid conditions. *Agents Actions,* **6,** 454–9
19. Dalziel, K., Going, C., Cartwright, P. H., Marks, R., Beveridge, G. W. and Rowell, N.R. (1986) Treatment of chronic discoid lupus erythematosus with an oral gold compound (auranofin). *Br. J. Dermatol.,* **115,** 211–6
20. Strömberg, H. E. and Ågren, M. S. (1984) Topical zinc oxide treatment improves arterial and venous leg ulcers. *Br. J. Dermatol.,* **111,** 461–8
21. Mohs, F. E. (1977) Chemosurgery for melanoma. *Arch. Dermatol.,* **113,** 285–91
22. Prasad, A.S., Miale, A. and Farid, Z. *et al* (1963) Biochemical studies on dwarfism, hypogonadism and anaemia. *Arch. Intern. Med.,* **111,** 407–8
23. Moynahan, E. J. and Barnes, P. M. (1973) Zinc deficiency and a synthetic diet for lactose intolerance. *Lancet,* **1,** 676–7
24. Michaelsson, G., Juhlin, L. and Vahlquist, A. (1977) Effects of oral zinc and vitamin A in acne. *Arch. Dermatol.,* **113,** 31–6
25. Wolowa, F. and Jablonska, S. (1978) Zinc sulphate in the treatment of alopecia areata. *Przegl. Dermatol.* (Warsaw), **65,** 687

26. Berne, B., Venge, P. and Ohman, S. (1985) Perifolliculitis Capitis Abscedens et Suffodiens (Hoffman). Complete healing associated with oral zinc therapy. *Arch. Dermatol.,* **121,** 1028–30
27. Mathur, N. K., Bumb, R. A. and Mangal, H. N. (1983) Zinc restores hair growth in lepromatous leprosy. *Br. J. Dermatol.,* **109,** 240
28. Sheard, C., Cormia, F. E. and Atkinson, S. C. (1957) Granulomatous reactions due to deodorant sticks. *J. Am. Med. Assoc.,* **164,** 1085–7

5

SKIN AND THE PSYCHE

J. A. COTTERILL

INTRODUCTION

There are psychological aspects in most patients presenting with skin disease. This is largely because the skin is a major organ in self-perception of body image and consequently any disturbance of the skin may lead to anxieties about body image, a lowering of self-esteem and in some patients, particularly with facial lesions, frank depression. Not only may skin disease result in anxiety or depression, but it may also be a presenting feature of an anxious, depressed, obsessional or frankly psychotic patient. It is important, therefore, that the dermatologist comes to recognize the dermatological presentations of these more serious psychiatric conditions. It is also important to remember that an increasing range of drugs used by a psychiatrist may produce skin disease and lithium-induced psoriasis and acne come readily to mind in this respect. Finally, the dermatologist will be called upon to deal with dermatological delusional disease, most often with a dysmorphophobic patient with a rich symptomatology referrable to the scalp, face and genital area. Fortunately the patient with delusions of parasitosis is much rarer.

BODY IMAGE AND DERMATOLOGICAL DISEASE

The concept of body image is partly perceptual, partly intellectual and totally abstract. Body image is largely cutaneous and the most important cutaneous areas in this percept include the hair, face – nose, eyes, mouth, breasts, especially in females, and genital area, especially in males. Every society modifies its body image in several fundamental ways. A common and acceptable way, especially in females, in our society, is by the use of cosmetics, shaving and hairstyling. More fundamental changes in body image can be made with the use and abuse of clothes, tattooing and scarification. What is desirable in terms of body image varies with time. Thus, in Victorian times, a pale, white, Dresden china-line skin was something to be treasured and prized. For instance, it is said that King Alphonso XIII of Spain insisted on black satin sheets on which to entertain his mistresses so that his white skin could be shown off to its best advantage. Whilst it is still desirable in northern and western Europe to have a bronzed skin, the pendulum may be swinging back towards Victorian times. President Reagan's nose may also be an important factor in this shift. It is also interesting that Miss World has become a progressively thinner, taller and less busty individual than she was in former times. The male-dominated advertising industry plays an important part in determining what women feel they should look like. The woman in 1987 is encouraged to be infantile about her skin. She is told in women's magazines that her skin needs 'feeding' and that it has to 'breathe', that cleansing is important, so she is exhorted to use a wide variety of 'baby' products on her skin. The desirable features for beauty are that skin should be spot and wrinkle-free, there should be no unpleasant odour and there should be no hair on the face, under the arms, on the legs, on the chest or abdomen, but plenty of hair on the head. The breasts should be so inconspicuous as to be almost nonexistent. In fact, the advertising machinery is telling the woman of 1987 that she should be prepubertal in her cutaneous desires. The gap that exists between these predominantly male-generated but feminine aspirations and reality can engender much cosmetic neurosis.

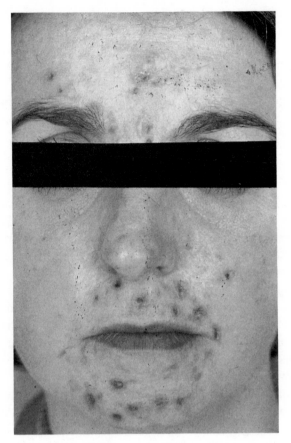

FIGURE 5.1   Acne excoriée

DERMATOLOGICAL DISORDERS AS A PRESENTING FEATURE OF PSYCHIATRIC DISTURBANCE

Acne excoriée des jeunes filles

Any teenager knows that there is a compelling instinct to pick and squeeze spots, but in acne excoriée this instinct is carried to an extreme. The patient, almost always a female, presents with excoriated lesions on the face, across the shoulders and occasionally in other body areas (Figure 5.1). This type of behaviour can be looked upon either as an exaggerated grooming response, or as a direct attack on the body image. It has been claimed that acne excoriée is a necessary protective device in patients with this disease[1]. If vigorous attempts are directed towards a cure, the skin disorder may be replaced by a frankly phobic patient. Thus acne excoriée is used to avoid painful life situations, which for most of the involved women means socialization, often concerning relationships with the opposite sex. If there is a real motivation on the part of the patient to be treated, trifluoperazine may be helpful in a small dosage, but usually it is important that the dermatologist does not cure the patient.

Neurodermatitis

Neurodermatitis may be localized or much more generalized. The areas of skin most affected by localized neurodermatitis or lichen simplex are the nape of the neck, especially in women, and the lateral aspects of the lower legs, especially in men. The extensor aspects of the forearm and around the elbows and lower back are also often involved. There are those who regard some forms of pruritus ani et vulvae as a localized form of neurodermatitis. In lichen simplex the skin becomes damaged by chronic scratching and in many patients this scratching and rubbing occurs whilst they are asleep in bed at night. Unless steps are taken to prevent this nocturnal scratching, the condition will persist.

Musaph has written about the 'traffic light phenomenon', claiming that short bursts of localized pruritus are a common manifestation of minor frustration from which the resultant scratching brings relief[2]. Musaph first noticed this phenomenon in motorists who are stopped at traffic lights. The minor frustration of being stopped produced itching and the resultant scratching resolved this frustration. In lichen simplex there may be an exaggeration of this mechanism and there is no doubt that some patients find scratching pleasurable. Indeed, some patients with chronic neurodermatitis develop very shiny, polished nails, preferring to rub rather than scratch.

With regard to management, the prevention of nocturnal scratching with an antihistamine or a short-acting benzodiazepine such as temazepam is often helpful. Local steroids often help to reduce the degree of pruritus. A small dose of superficial X-ray is often helpful, particularly in isolated lesions of lichen simplex on the posterior neck or lateral shins. Occlusive therapy may be helpful too, particularly on the legs or on the arms. All these measures help cut across the itch/scratch cycle. It is also important to talk to the patient to try and establish any factors which may be causing stress or conflict. Any accompanying significant anxiety or depression should be treated accordingly.

Generalized pruritus

It is true to say that in the vast majority of patients no organic cause for generalized pruritus is found and in this situation it is commonplace for dermatologists to attribute the itching to psychological factors, often on very ill-founded grounds. It is important to investigate any patient presenting with generalized pruritus to rule out any significant underlying disease and the most useful investigations, after a full history and examination, in such a work-up include liver function tests, a full blood count, urea, serum iron, serum calcium and thyroid function tests. There is no doubt that generalized pruritus may be stress and conflict-induced in some patients, but it is unusual for the patient to link this symptomatology to his problems.

Dermatitis artefacta[3,4]

Self-induced dermatological lesions are seen most commonly in female patients between the age of 10–20 years. In this situation it is usually relatively easy to determine the upsetting factors in the patient's environment and often remedy these, which results in a complete cure. Lesions of artefact dermatitis tend to occur in patients with an angry, hysterical type of personality typified by Florence Nightingale. It is therefore interesting that there may be an association between the desire to nurse and the desire to be nursed and indeed, artefact dermatitis is not unusual in nurses or paramedical staff, particularly if they are not succeeding well. There are several clues to diagnosis. The lesions are usually bizarre and in accessible positions on the skin. They may have very straight or unusual circular edges. Damage is always most marked on the upper part of the skin, becoming less with increasing inward depth and this can be shown readily histologically.

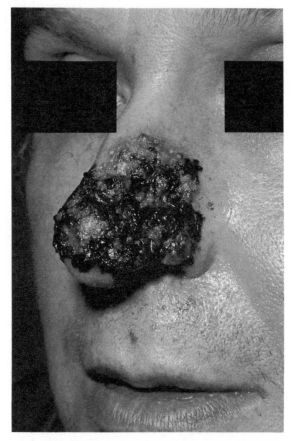

FIGURE 5.2   Dermatitis artefacta

The lesions heal very rapidly with simple nursing measures such as occlusive bandaging. The patients seem to have a 'belle indifférence' to the symptomatology and may reassure the doctor and tell him not to worry. All the lesions are fully developed and no lesions are seen in various states of evolution. There is usually a 'hollow' history and the patient cannot describe the evolution of an individual lesion.

Whilst artefact dermatitis in a young female carries a relatively good prognosis, artefact dermatitis occurring in older patients carries a much more ominous prognosis. In older men, artefact dermatitis may be associated with attempts at industrial compensation, whereas in

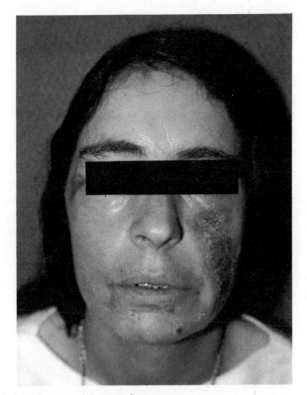

FIGURE 5.3 Dermatitis artefacta

older women it is often associated with refractory depression or frank psychosis, such as schizophrenia.

The morphology of artefact lesions varies enormously (Figures 5.2, 5.3, 5.4). Isolated blisters are a common presentation in young females. A very crusted lesion which heals relatively rapidly should alert physicians' suspicions. In older females, artefact dermatitis may be just one part of a wide spectrum of simulated disease and the medical notes of such a patient may be very thick. This is another clue to diagnosis. In younger patients the commonest precipitating factors involve difficulty in communication with the parents, usually the mother, marital problems, housing problems, problems at school and problems with boyfriends. The lesion may be used to manipulate the parents and I have seen artefact dermatitis used to persuade parents

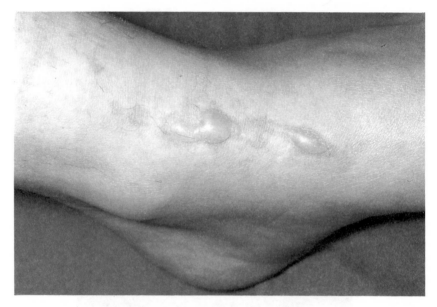

FIGURE 5.4   Dermatitis artefacta on the ankle

to buy a young female a horse, and on another occasion to avoid being sent away to school.

It is thought to be important not to confront the patient with the fact that the lesion is known to be self-induced. I usually tell the patient that in my view the lesion has arisen because the skin has been in contact with something noxious in the patient's environment. I usually say that I don't know what this agent is, but that I have seen this situation before and in a young female and I reassure both the parents and the child that this situation will eventually disappear. It is important to explore problems with the child's parents. The problems are usually quite superficial and amenable to relatively simple solutions. It is also important not just to discharge the patient as soon as the lesions do disappear, so that the patient learns that they can come to see a sympathetic dermatologist without any cutaneous offerings. If this course of action is followed, it is usually not long before the patient defaults from follow-up. The older female patient with artefact dermatitis is an insoluble problem and psychiatrists are not very anxious to get involved.

Trichotillomania

The psychodynamics of trichotillomania (Figure 5.5) are very similar to those of artefact dermatitis. Below the age of five, male children predominate, but after this age trichotillomania is a predominantly female pursuit. The prognosis is good in young females below the age of 20, but in the older female the prognosis is poor and is usually associated with frank psychiatric disease, such as significant depression or anxiety states. Trichotillomania may follow a bereavement, particularly of a brother or sister or of one parent, and may be seen as part of marital disharmony and as a result of poor housing and difficulties at school[5,6]. In the young female with trichotillomania the problem is usually fairly easy to resolve. In a child under five years it may be more difficult to treat. Child psychiatrists often arm the child with a little artificial hair to play with to try and persuade them to play with this rather than their own hair. Spock has pointed out that most babies play and fiddle with their hair anyway and trichotillomania again can be looked upon as an exaggeration of a normal grooming response.

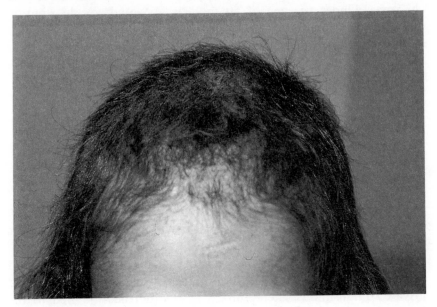

FIGURE 5.5   Trichotillomania

DERMATOLOGICAL DELUSIONAL DISEASE

The best-known form of dermatological delusional disease is delusion of parasitosis, but this condition is exceedingly rare. Much more common are those dysmorphophobic patients with dermatological non-disease, who have delusions or overvalued ideas involving the scalp, face, including the mouth, and genital area.

Delusions of parasitosis

Lyell[7] has made some detailed studies of this condition. A personal survey of dermatologists in the UK revealed only 285 cases. It was apparent from this study that the classical patient with delusions of parasitosis tends to be socially isolated and often eccentric. Lyell makes the point that it is often difficult to know where eccentricity ends and madness begins. The patients are usually intelligent and the professions were well represented in Lyell's survey. The medical profession is also well represented, particularly in the form of psychiatrists. Under the age of 50 there is an equal sex distribution and frank psychiatric disease, either in the form of schizophrenia or depression, shared delusions or drug addiction may be present. Over the age of 50 women predominate 3:1 and bereavement may be a triggering factor. Depression is quite common.

Clinical features

The patient presents with a complaint that they are infested with parasites and this claim is usually substantiated with a wide variety of specimens collected from the scalp or other body areas and usually presented in a small box or plastic packet (Figure 5.6). The patient is often very tired because of excessive washing and housecleaning. Shared delusions with other members of the family are quite common (folie à deux, à trois etc.). The local authority disinfestation centre or private organisations like Rentokil have often been invited to the house to deal with the alleged problem. Samples may have been sent

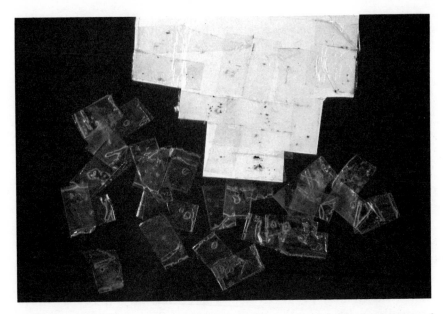

FIGURE 5.6 Sellotaped packets from a patient with delusions of parasitosis

to the local university or farther afield to such places as the British Museum.

From a psychiatric point of view the predominant disturbance present is usually one of primary monosymptomatic hypochondriacal psychosis[8]. Munro defined this condition as a disorder characterized by a single hypochondriacal delusional system, relatively distinct from the remainder of the personality. The delusion may be accompanied by illusional misperceptions, or at times possibly by ill-defined hallucinations. Munro stressed that in monosymptomatic hypochondriacal psychosis the rest of the personality is relatively unaffected by the psychotic process and so the patient is able to communicate absolutely normally on all other topics[8]. However, about half the patients are also significantly depressed and in some patients there may be features of both primary monosymptomatic hypochondriacal psychosis and depression. The possibility of drug addiction must not be forgotten, especially in a younger patient.

Management of patients with delusions of parasitosis

The management of a typical patient with delusions of parasitosis is never easy and by the time a patient is referred to the dermatologist the emotional temperature of the whole family is usually very high. In my opinion it is best to admit the patient, who will usually agree to this procedure. This manœuvre also gives other family members some relief from the constant anxieties engendered over the 'parasites' by the index patient. Lyell[7] has stressed that some patients with delusions of parasitosis have underlying organic disease and a full history, examination and investigations along the lines of those done for patients with generalized pruritus is mandatory.

If there is no evidence of any underlying organic disease and the patient appears to have just one isolated delusion in an otherwise clear blue sky, a therapeutic trial of pimozide is indicated. The initial dose is 2 mg and this is best given in a single morning dose as in some individuals it may produce sleeplessness. The dose may need to be gradually increased up to a maximum of 8–12 mg daily, but on higher doses extrapyramidal symptoms often become prominent. One side-effect of treatment is depression and it is thought this may be analogous to the depression which may occur during the recovery stages of other forms of psychosis. At this stage an antidepressant may be required. Unfortunately, compliance is poor and usually as soon as therapy is stopped the delusions reappear. In this group of patients a weekly depot injection of fluspirilene, a parenteral analogue of pimozide, can be given. In my experience, most patients with delusions of parasitosis are readily lost to follow-up. In patients where depression seems to be a dominant feature clinically, there may be a good response to treatment with antidepressants alone.

DYSMORPHOPHOBIA IN DERMATOLOGICAL NON-DISEASE

Every dermatologist sees a relatively large number of patients, predominantly female, presenting with no objective skin pathology on examination, but with a rich dermatological symptomatology. Symptomatology is referred to three main body areas, namely the face and mouth, scalp and perineum. Symptomatology referrable to face, mouth and scalp are much more common in females than males, whereas genital symptomatology is much more common in males than females.

Presenting symptoms

The most common symptomatology referrable to the face is a complaint of burning and it is important to remember that very few dermatological conditions are able to produce this symptom. Light eruptions, including forms of porphyria, are a notable exception where a burning feeling may be experienced. However, in the vast majority of patients presenting with the symptom of burning, the aetiology is functional. Other facial symptoms include a concern over excessive facial hair, excessively large pores, the shape of the nose and imagined scarring or redness. Patients may also present with persistent pain in the mouth or located to the tongue (orodynia, glossodynia). This discomfort is unremitting or may become worse towards the end of the day. Scalp symptomatology includes a complaint of severe burning and of excessive hair loss. Presenting symptoms in the genital area include severe discomfort, making it difficult to sit down. Male patients are more common in this group, which also consists of generally older patients. Symptoms may follow genuine or imagined exposure to venereal infection, often many years previously. Others may present with a complaint that the scrotum is burning and red and there may be an associated discomfort on the upper anterior thighs, which is made worse by contact with clothes. A feeling that there is excessive redness of the foreskin or of the skin of the shaft of the penis may also be of concern and venereologists see patients who are convinced they have a significant urethral discharge.

Vulvodynia is the non-disease equivalent in females. The severe intractable pain in the vulval area has a devastating effect on marriage and on the quality of life of the patient. Some women with this disorder are unable to sit or go to bed because of the discomfort. In a significant proportion of patients this type of symptomatology arises after surgery, and particularly after gynaecological operations such as hysterectomy or vulvectomy.

97

Psychiatric aspects

The most common psychiatric disease present is depression[9], although patients with senile dementia, schizophrenia and obsessional neurosis may all present to the dermatologist with this type of symptomatology. The depression is severe enough, particularly in female patients with facial disease, to make them try and commit suicide, sometimes successfully. This may be done in a rather dramatic way, for instance, by the use of petrol poured over the body or even by standing in front of a moving railway train.

Other clinical features[10]

There are often difficulties in making suitable appointments with patients who usually want to be seen urgently. Urgent appointments are often cancelled at the last minute and then remade at short notice. The consultation with the patient with non-disease always takes much longer than a patient with organic disease and even after the consultation the patient may constantly telephone the doctor for further advice and assurance. Once seen, most patients with dermatological non-disease like to be seen frequently for follow-up purposes. The referral letter from the patient's family doctor is often much longer than that sent with a patient with organic disease and the dermatologist may respond also with a longer letter than he is accustomed to write. Patients with dermatological non-disease do not take well to a snap decision to refer them to a psychiatrist. The importance of a liaison clinic in a department of dermatology is underlined by this situation. Unhappily, also, some psychiatrists are not very familiar with the management of dysmorphophobic patients.

Management

As a group, dysmorphophobic patients with dermatological non-disease fail to respond to a wide range of either topical or oral therapy and a placebo response is never seen. Often, however, a nocebo response is characteristic in that the patient will develop symptomatology when given a placebo. Although many patients with dermatological non-disease are significantly depressed, their response to antidepressants is poor. They usually say they sleep better, but their delusions or overvalued ideas tend to persist. Within this group of patients there are those who are either anxiously preoccupied or have an overvalued idea about their physical characteristics and this may be a presenting feature of emotional problems, such as matrimonial problems or financial problems at home or at work. This group of patients will often do quite well with relatively superficial psychotherapy.

IDIOPATHIC OEDEMA OF WOMEN

Idiopathic, cyclical or periodic oedema is an ill-understood condition, occurring almost exclusively in females and characterized by episodes of fluid retention. Classically patients show a daily weight gain of at least 1.4 kg and in some cases the diurnal weight increase may be as much as 6 kg. There is never any underlying heart, kidney or liver disease or lymphatic or venous obstruction. Patients presenting with this disorder complain of swelling of the face, fingers, hands, abdomen and legs which becomes progressively worse as the day goes on. More important than the swelling, many patients develop psychiatric disturbances and the incidence of divorce is very high. Depression, anxiety, hysteria and true psychosis have all been described. The personality of affected patients has been described as shrewish and abrasive. In some patients this type of symptomatology has followed laxative or diuretic abuse and it has been suggested that a hypothalamic lesion may predispose to not only the psychiatric aspects of the disorder, but also induce the endocrine changes which lead to sodium and water retention.

Management of the patient with periodic oedema

Management of patients with this condition is not easy. The entity often goes unrecognized by physician colleagues and patients are often reassured when a firm diagnosis can be given for their problems. It is important to persuade the patient to stop smoking as this leads to fluid retention and salt restriction in the diet is also helpful. The use of diuretics is controversial. There may be a place for tranquillizers in the anxious patient and antidepressants for the depressed patient. Although the disorder may persist for years it sometimes does remit spontaneously[11].

References

1. Sneddon, J., Sneddon, I. B. (1983). Acne excoriée: a protective device. *Clin. Exp. Dermatol.*, **8**, 65–8
2. Musaph, H. (1983). Psychogenic pruritus. *Semin. Dermatol.*, **2**, 217–22
3. Sneddon, I., Sneddon, J. (1975). Self-inflicted injury: a follow-up study of 43 patients. *Br. Med. J.*, **3**, 527–30
4. Sneddon, I. B. (1983). Simulated disease and hypochondriasis in the dermatology clinic. *Semin. Dermatol.*, **2**, 177–81
5. Cotterill, J. A. (1985). The psychosomatics of trichotillomania. *Dermatologica*, **171**, 498
6. Oranje, A. P., Teereboom-Wynia, J. D. R. & Raeymaecker, D. M. J. de (1986). Trichotillomania in childhood. *J. Am. Acad. Dermatol.*, **15**, 614–19
7. Lyell, A. (1983). Delusions of parasitosis. *Semin. Dermatol.*, **2**, 189–95
8. Munro, A. (1983). Delusional parasitosis: a form of monosymptomatic hypochondriacal psychosis. *Semin. Dermatol.*, **2**, 197–202
9. Cotterill, J. A. (1981). Dermatological non-disease: a common and potentially fatal disturbance in cutaneous body image. *Br. J. Dermatol.*, **104**, 611–18
10. Cotterill, J. A. (1983). Clinical features of patients with dermatological non-disease. *Semin. Dermatol.*, **2**, 203–5
11. Pelosi, A. J., Lough, J. R., Sykes, R. A., Muir, W. J. and Dunnigan, M. G. (1986). A psychiatric study of idiopathic oedema. *Lancet*, **2**, 999–1001

Index

87/11

SCHOOLS COUNCIL

MODULAR COURSES IN TECHNOLOGY

MATERIALS
TECHNOLOGY

John McShea

David Byrne

Kenneth Danks

Terry Hewitt

Norman Wooley

Oliver & Boyd

in association with the National Centre for School Technology

PROJECT TEAM

Director
Dr Ray Page

Co-ordinators
Roy Pickup
John Poole

Jeffrey Hall
Dr Duncan Harris
John Hucker
Michael Ive
Peter Patient

Oliver & Boyd
Robert Stevenson House
1–3 Baxter's Place
Leith Walk
Edinburgh EH1 3BB

A Division of Longman Group UK Ltd

ISBN 0-05-003395-6

First published 1981
Fifth impression 1986

Produced by Longman Group (FE) Ltd
Printed in Hong Kong

Contents

Acknowledgments

For permission to reproduce certain photographs in this book, the authors and publishers would like to thank the following:

The Controller of Her Majesty's Stationery Office (Fig. 1);

The Trustees of the British Museum (Fig. 2);

The Central Electricity Generating Board (Fig. 1.1);

The Electricity Council (Fig. 1.3);

NASA (Figs. 1.4 and 1.5);

G. Maunsell & Partners (Fig. 1.6);

ICI Plastics Division (Figs. 1.8, 6.6, 6.13, 6.17, 6.19, 6.22 and 6.25);

The *New Civil Engineer* (Fig. 1.12);

Freeman Fox & Partners and William Tribe Ltd (Fig. 1.13);

Keystone Press Agency Ltd (Fig. 1.14);

Dr T. N. Baker and the Department of Metallurgy at Strathclyde University (Figs. 2.10 and 2.11);

British Steel Corporation (Fig. 3.1);

RTZ Services Ltd (Figs. 3.2, 5.1 and 5.11);

National Machinery GmbH, Nuernberg (Fig. 4.2);

TI (Group services) Ltd (Fig. 4.3, from the paper 'Moiré patterns on electron micrographs and their applications to the study of dislocations in metals' by G. A. Bassett, J. W. Menter and D. W. Pashley, published in Proceedings of the Royal Society, A, Vol. 246, p. 345);

BCIRA (Figs. 5.3 and 5.4);

Birmal Castings Ltd (Figs. 5.5 and 5.6);

The Firth Derihon Stampings Ltd (Figs. 5.7 and 5.8);

GKN Bound Brook Ltd (Fig. 5.10);

Scandinavian Aluminium Profiles AB Ltd (Fig. 5.12);

Griffin & George Ltd (Figs. 5.13 and 5.17);

EPS Association (Fig. 6.3);

British Industrial Plastics Ltd (Figs. 6.10, 6.11, 6.12 and 6.14);

Shell (UK) Ltd (Fig. 6.20);

The Malaysian Rubber Producers' Research Association Photographic Unit (Figs. 7.1 and 7.4a);

Dunlop Ltd (Figs. 7.2, 7.3, 7.4b and c).

Preface

This book will show you the importance of materials to our way of life. Because we live in what is called a 'high technology' society, materials play an increasingly important part in determining our personal standard of living and the overall prosperity of the country. This book will bring to your attention not only the everyday appliances which make life more comfortable, but also some of the more sophisticated needs of industry. You will hear the following questions asked more and more frequently.

Can we afford to live in a high technology society?

What will happen when the energy resources for producing materials run out?

How can we use materials more efficiently?

If we have to reduce our consumption of materials, which, if any, could we afford to do without?

These questions will have to be answered in your lifetime. As the Third World continues to develop industrially, the same share of the world's dwindling energy and material sources is no longer available only to rich countries. In simple terms, our slice of the energy/materials cake is getting smaller and smaller. What will you be able to do about it? A knowledge of materials is essential to any real understanding of modern technology. With knowledge we can plan for the future with understanding.

The sign ■ has been used to signify material suitable for both O-level and CSE candidates. The sign □ indicates material suitable for O-level candidates only.

Introduction

■ The Development of Materials

Energy and materials are the basic resources of mankind. It is understandable therefore that early history uses the names of materials to describe the important stages of our development, e.g. the Stone Age, Bronze Age and Iron Age. It was the discovery of metals which allowed us to construct the tools and weapons with which to survive.

The time scale of such developments varied considerably between different continents, depending on the ease with which the metals were discovered or extracted. Some civilisations were in a Bronze Age while others, who possibly had less resources, were still in a Stone Age.

We are apt to consider early civilisations as very primitive but in fact their skills were well developed for the tools at their disposal, and some of their techniques have never been improved upon.

In England, for example, work on Stonehenge was started around 2000 BC and consisted of a simple ring of stones. The final period in the construction commenced around 1600 BC and we can still see the remains of this today (Fig. 1a). In Fig. 1b you can see the tenon at the top of the upright, and the mortise on the underside of the lintel. These were used to key the blocks together. This method of construction was achieved by pounding the rock with heavy stone hammers.

Fig. 1 Stonehenge   (a)   (b)

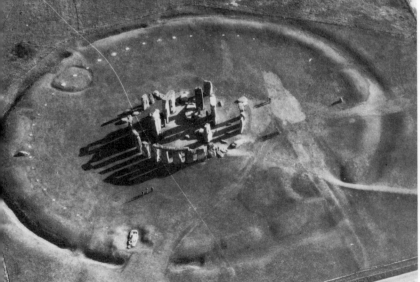
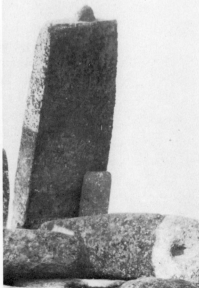

By this time (the early Bronze Age), tools and weapons of bronze and ornaments of gold were being made in Ireland and traded across Britain to the continent.

In the Middle East (Egypt and Sumeria), metals had been worked since around 8000 BC. The metals were those which occurred naturally, such as gold and copper. Being soft, they could be beaten into shape easily and were much valued as ornaments. The ability to extract copper from the copper-bearing ore, malachite, was common in the East. Copper in fact derives its name from the island of Cyprus where there were mines as early as 3000 BC.

Unworked copper is a soft metal and was of only limited use for tools. When melted together with tin it formed an **alloy** called bronze, which was found to be much harder and more suitable for tools and weapons. When two or more metals are melted together to form a new metal, it is called an alloy. The process is called **alloying** and is used to improve the properties of the original metals.

Fig. 2   A beaten bronze shield (known as the Battersea shield) from the early Iron Age in Britain

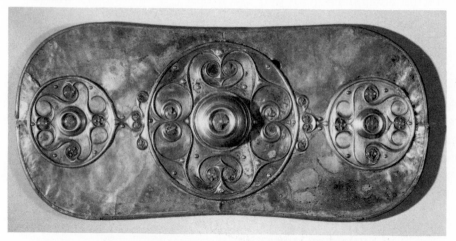

In Europe, it was not long before bronze was superseded by iron. Although iron from meteorites had been used earlier, it was not until around 1400 BC that iron was obtained from its ore, haematite. The Hittite people, who established an empire in Turkey and Syria, made their weapons from iron. These weapons were made by hammering iron after heating it with charcoal. Heating iron in this way causes it to absorb carbon from the charcoal and form an alloy called steel. The collapse of the Hittite empire around 1200 BC was largely responsible for spreading the knowledge of this process.

As surface deposits of ore were used up, people began to mine and in time they became more proficient at extracting the metals and alloying them.

By the Middle Ages primitive blast furnaces were in operation and in the next few hundred years various improvements in the process were carried out.

Then, in 1709, Abraham Darby introduced the use of coked coal as a furnace fuel in the production of iron (coke is coal which has been heated carefully in the absence of air to remove impurities such as sulphur). Coke is able to support the heavy weight of ore inside a furnace and large quantities of iron could be produced at one time.

In 1845 aluminium was isolated from its ore, bauxite, by Friedrich Wöhler. Its scarcity in metallic form made it very valuable, and Napoleon III of France used to boast of his aluminium dinner service.

In 1856 it was Henry Bessemer who finally developed a method of producing large quantities of cheap steel. Molten iron was transferred to a **converter** in which the carbon content of the steel could be carefully controlled. This method is still used in modern blast furnaces.

The first commercial plastic, Parkesine, was developed by Alexander Parkes, a metallurgist who was interested in materials which were easy to mould into complex shapes. The material was first displayed in London at the International Exhibition of 1862. Although Parkesine was not a successful material it paved the way for the development of modern plastics. In the twentieth century there have been many exciting developments in these materials and they are as important as metals to an advanced technological society.

The exploitation of materials has provided the tools which have enabled us to progress. The challenge of modern technology is not only to make use of new materials but to make more efficient and imaginative use of those already established.

1 The Properties of Materials

■ Introduction

An engineer or designer, when considering the solution to a design problem, must have a thorough knowledge of the properties of any material which may influence its particular use. This knowledge allows him to select a suitable material from the vast range at his disposal. Within his solution, the engineer must ensure a high level of operational safety, particularly where human life is at risk, high standards of manufacture, the satisfactory appearance of the finished article and allow for the economics of production and marketing. It is through a detailed knowledge of materials and their properties that the engineer/designer achieves these aims.

Understanding the process of selecting a material for a particular design function, from the vast range available, can be simplified by grouping them into metals and non-metals. This simple grouping is one way of emphasising the properties of materials, but is not the strict chemical division of metallic and non-metallic elements.

■ Electrical Conductivity

At various levels all materials resist the flow of electricity. Electrical **conductors** are those materials which offer a very low level of resistance to the flow of electricity.

The metals are good electrical conductors, though some are better than others. Copper, one of the best, is used in cables for supplying electricity to power points around the house, or to machines in industry

However, without varying levels of resistance it would be difficult to operate everyday household appliances such as toasters and electric fires. The electricity flowing in the copper transmission wire from the plug to the machine creates little heat. The reason for this is the very low resistance of copper. Nichrome, an alloy of nickel and chromium, is used in the form of a thin wire to produce the desired high resistance for use as a heating element.

In order to make the best use of electrical conductors, we must be able to insulate the electricity for safety reasons. An electrical **insulator** is a material which offers a very high level of resistance to the flow of electricity. Non-metals are generally good insulators, but all insulators vary in their ability to resist electricity.

Wood is a comparatively poor insulator whilst ceramic materials (pottery)

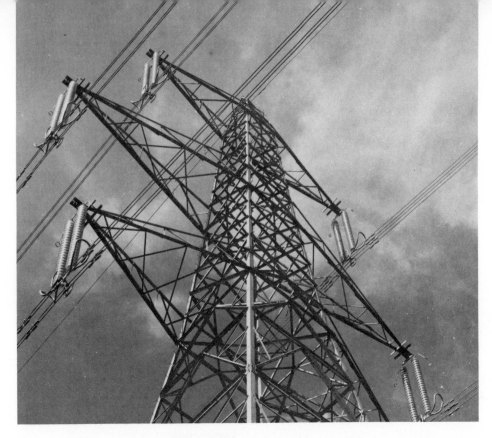

Fig. 1.1   Ceramic insulators supporting cables from an electricity pylon

are very good. Ceramic insulators are used to isolate power cables from the pylons carrying them (Fig. 1.1), and in rod form are also used in electric fires to support the heating element. Mica in sheet form finds similar use in electric toasters.

☐ Semiconductors

Between the two extremes of good conductors and good insulators, are materials which allow an electric current to flow only under certain conditions. Such materials are known as semi-conductors, and silicon and germanium are examples of these.

In their pure state, silicon and germanium are poor conductors of electricity but their electrical resistance can be altered by careful addition of tiny quantities of selected materials introduced as 'impurities'. Devices such as

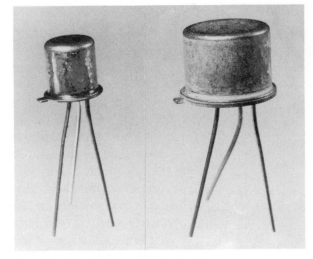

Fig. 1.2   Transistors—an example of the use of semiconductor materials

transistors are produced from semiconductor materials. The resistance of semiconductors can be considerably affected by heat and light energy. This means that they can be used to sense a change in thermal conditions or in the intensity of light. This property is widely used in such devices as fire alarms, light meters for cameras, etc.

■ Thermal Conductivity

'Therm' is an ancient Greek word for heat. It is often met as part of other words, e.g. thermometer, thermostat, thermos flask. Thermal conductivity relates to heat and how heat travels through a material. It is measured in watts per metre degree Celsius.

Metals are all good conductors of heat although some are better than others. We use metal hot-plates on cookers to conduct the heat from the electric element to the saucepan. The metal saucepan then conducts this heat to the food.

From the list of values of thermal conductivities, can you explain why car radiator fins are made of copper rather than steel?

Thermal Conductivity (W/m°C)

Metals		Non-metals	
Copper	386	Graphite	150
Aluminium	200	Pyrex glass	1.2
Brass	120	Soda-lime glass	0.8
Steel	55	Polyethylene	0.3
Invar	11	Rubber	0.1
		Concrete	0.1
		Polyurethane foam	0.05

Thermal insulators are those materials with a low value of thermal conductivity. In general, non-metals are thermal insulators and are used to prevent heat gains or losses. Kettles, saucepans and irons have plastic or wood handles to prevent the heat being conducted from the hot metal to your hands. Notable exceptions to the use of non-metals as insulators are ceramic dishes, such as Pyrex, and the ceramic hob cooking stove.

Thermal insulators are also used to reduce heat losses in the home. Air is one of the best thermal insulators and materials which trap air have been specially devised. Glass fibre matting is used to insulate lofts, and formaldehyde foam to insulate cavity walls in houses. Refrigerator casings are insulated with polyurethane foam to keep heat out.

The demands of space technology are particularly exacting. During re-entry, the surface temperature of a spacecraft can reach about 1500°C, so virtually the whole surface of the light alloy structure has to be insulated or it would melt

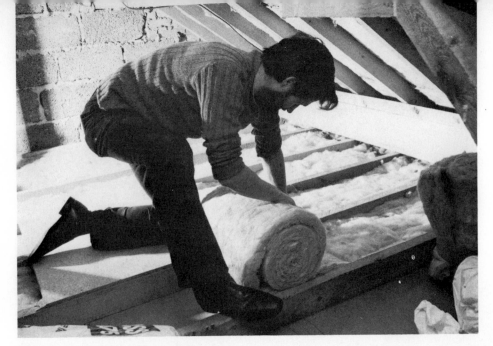

Fig. 1.3   Laying glass fibre roof insulation

and vapourise. In the Apollo command modules the material used was a mixture of asbestos, glass fibre and nylon. The protective heat shield gradually disintegrated, forming a protective layer of gas or liquid which was continually swept away, thus cooling the module by evaporation. The shield was thick enough to ensure that it was not completely burnt away during re-entry. However, such modules are not re-usable. The re-usable space shuttle has been designed with graphite panels to insulate the hottest leading areas, and silica tiles to protect the cabin. These panels can be replaced if necessary.

Fig. 1.4   The scorched protective shield of an Apollo command module

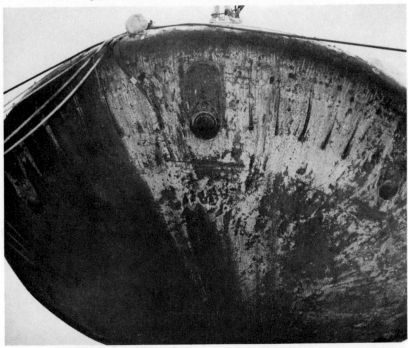

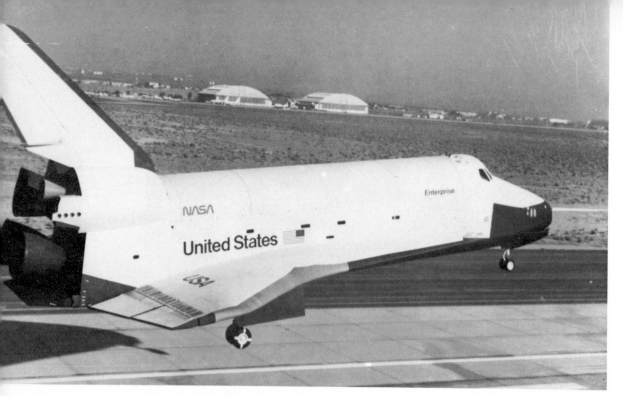

Fig. 1.5   The space shuttle Orbiter 101 'Enterprise' coming in to land after a test flight

■ Thermal Expansion

With few exceptions, materials expand as they get hot and shrink as they cool down. The coefficient of linear expansion of a material is the fractional change in length caused by change in temperature. This is a number and not a unit of measurement. The table shows the widely different thermal expansions of a variety of materials.

Coefficients of Linear Expansion/°C

Polyurethane foam	0.000 090
Rubber	0.000 670
Polyethylene	0.000 300
Aluminium	0.000 025
Brass	0.000 019
Copper	0.000 018
Steel	0.000 012
Concrete	0.000 011
Soda-lime glass	0.000 009
Pyrex glass	0.000 003
Graphite	0.000 002
Invar	0.000 001

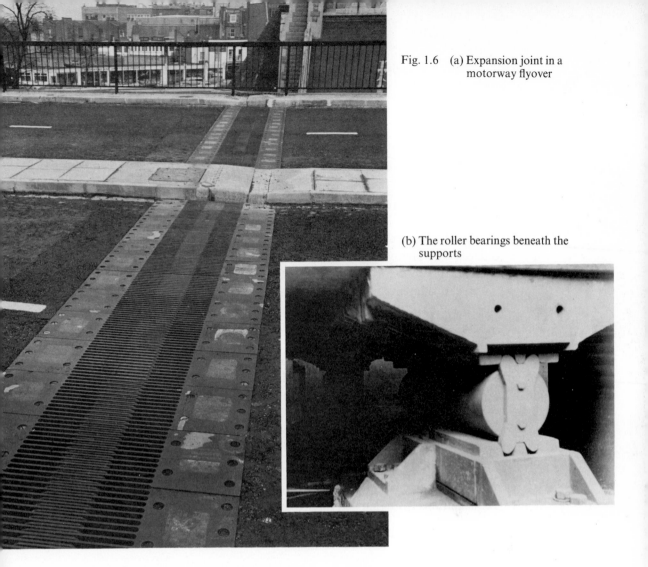

Fig. 1.6   (a) Expansion joint in a motorway flyover

(b) The roller bearings beneath the supports

The seasonal variations in temperature are sufficient to cause appreciable thermal movements in large structures, a factor which a civil engineer has to consider in the design of a bridge. You have probably observed the expansion joints in the road surfaces of bridges, and the rollers beneath the end supports, which assist this movement. Without adequate provision for expansion, the road would crack or buckle.

Thermal movement can, however, be used to advantage, particularly where it is necessary to monitor temperature changes. The bimetallic strip in a heat-sensitive switch is designed to give a significant mechanical movement when a small change in temperature occurs. A strip of brass is bonded to a strip of Invar and clamped at one end. Since brass expands considerably more than Invar, a change in temperature will cause the bimetallic strip to bend appreciably. This movement can be used as a control mechanism.

Can you suggest why Invar is used in a bimetallic strip?

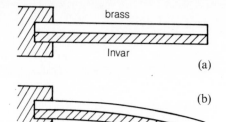

(a)

(b)

Fig. 1.7   A bimetallic strip
(a) Before heating   (b) After heating

Bimetallic strips are frequently used to open and close electrical circuits. An application of this is in thermostats to activate central-heating systems in the home and industry. A thermostat is a switch or valve which is operated or controlled by changes in temperature. A control dial allows the thermostat to be manually altered to switch at the desired temperature.

Some automatic kettles are controlled by a bimetallic strip. The steam from boiling water directed over the strip, causes subsequent expansion and releases a set of electrical contacts which break the circuit.

A car thermostat acts as a valve to regulate the flow of water to the engine. When the engine is cold, the valve isolates the water in the engine block from the main supply of cooling water in the radiator. The water in the block heats up quite quickly as does the engine, and this ensures fuel economy and improved performance as well as reducing wear. As the engine approaches its normal working temperature, the bimetallic mechanism in the thermostat gradually opens the valve, allowing the circulation of an increasing volume of cooling water to maintain the engine at its optimum temperature.

☐ **Calculations Involving Thermal Expansion**

To calculate the thermal expansion of a length of material, the following equation is used:

change in length = coefficient of linear expansion × original length ×
change in temperature.

Example
A 5 m length of PVC plumbing waste pipe is installed along the external wall of a house when the temperature is 20°C. If the coefficient of thermal expansion of PVC is 13×10^{-5}, calculate the contraction that will take place when the temperature drops to 0°C.

Contraction = coefficient of linear expansion × original length ×
drop in temperature
$$= 13 \times 10^{-5} \times 5 \times 20$$
$$= 1300 \times 10^{-5}$$
$$= 0.013 \, \text{m}$$
i.e. the pipe is reduced in length by 0.013 m.

16

■ Optical Properties

These properties deal with the way in which materials react to light. Most metals are good reflectors of light if polished. Reflectors are used in car headlamps and as mirrors. Metals also have very distinctive colours, and this, combined with their reflective properties, makes them easily recognisable.

The optical properties of non-metals vary considerably. Wood, which is normally opaque, can be cut thin enough to make it translucent, whilst glass is completely transparent. The biggest users of glass are of course the building and related industries. Other materials like acrylic may be transparent and are finding more frequent application where their optical properties are enhanced by other factors such as their reduced weight.

Colour is another important optical feature and this is often modified by using pigments in paints or dyes. For instance, cameras require internal metal surfaces that are totally non-reflective and matt black paints have to be used.

The colour of a surface also determines to a certain extent its ability to absorb or radiate heat. Thus in a solar panel, used to provide hot water or heat for a building, the pipes or channels are black to absorb the most heat from the sun.

Fig. 1.8   Solar panels used to heat a swimming pool

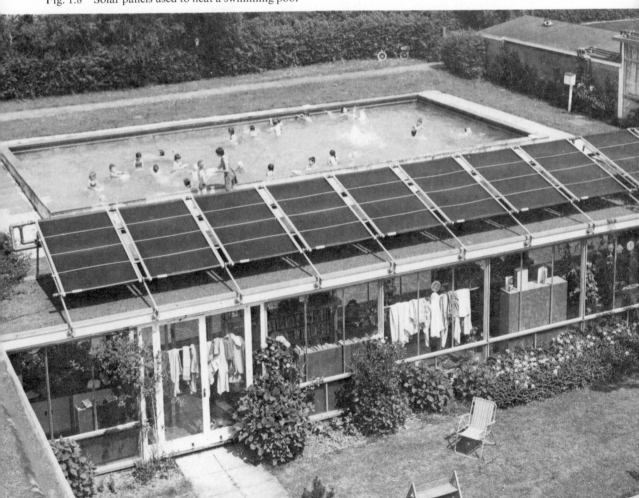

■ Magnetic Properties

That magnetism can be used as a force is clearly seen by the attraction of the unlike poles of a pair of magnets, and the repulsion of like poles. Whenever electricity flows in a wire, a magnetic field is produced.

This can be observed by passing a current through a length of wire and placing the wire parallel to the needle of a compass, which will be deflected. The direction of movement of the needle depends upon the direction of the current flow in the wire.

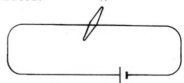

Fig. 1.9   The magnetic effect of a current

This relationship between electricity and magnetism is known as the electromagnetic effect. When a length of wire wrapped round a soft iron core is connected to a battery, we call it an electromagnet because it acts as a magnet when an electric current flows through the wire.

Whenever you use a telephone, radio, television or record player, you are making use of the electromagnetic effect to operate a loudspeaker. Varying electrical signals from the equipment are received by a coil of wire known as the speech coil of the loudspeaker. The changing magnetic field produced by this coil causes it to be moved by the surrounding magnet. The paper or aluminium diaphragm connected to the speech coil moves a column of air to produce sound waves.

The electricity flowing through the armature coil of an electric motor creates a magnetic field, the moving force being provided by a second magnetic field fixed around the armature.

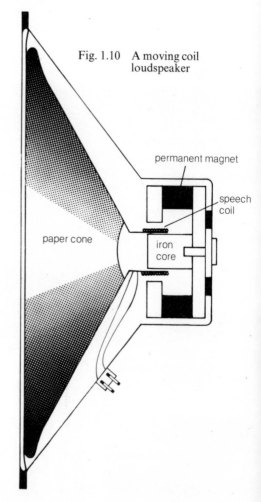

Fig. 1.10   A moving coil loudspeaker

permanent magnet

speech coil

paper cone

iron core

Fig. 1.11   A simple electric motor

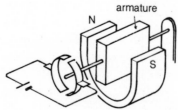

armature

N

S

A commutator, consisting of a split metal ring, allows the rotating armature to break electrical contact with the supply and remake it with the current flowing in the opposite direction. The change in direction of current reverses the direction of the magnetic field and allows the rotation to continue.

In a similar way, a generator converts rotational motion into electrical energy by moving a coil through a fixed magnetic field.

■ Mechanical Properties

When a material is subjected to a sufficiently high force it will deform in one of two ways, either elastically or plastically.

(a) **Elastic** deformation describes the ability of a material to return to its original shape and size after this force has been removed. A pneumatic tyre is a common example of the property of elasticity.

(b) **Plastic** deformation describes the ability of a material to remain permanently deformed even after the force has been removed. This property of plasticity allows materials to be pressed into a new shape which they will retain. Red-hot steel has good plasticity.

Metals which are able to deform extensively before fracture are said to be **ductile**. The ductility of metals is an important property which enables sheet metal articles to be pressed into deep shapes such as car body panels, kitchen sinks, etc.

Conversely those materials which exhibit little or no deformation before fracture are said to be **brittle**. Window glass is an example of a brittle material.

Toughness is the property which indicates the amount of energy that can be absorbed by a material. Trying to break off the lid of a tin can by bending it backwards and forwards is remarkably difficult because steel is a tough metal.

The **strength** of a material is a measure of its ability to withstand mechanical deformation. There are three common ways of deforming a material.

(a) **Tension** is a pulling force. You have to apply a tensile force when you use a catapult.

(b) **Compression** is a squeezing force. The legs of your chair are in compression due to your weight which applies a compressive force.

(c) **Torsion** is a twisting force. The use of a screwdriver demands the application of forces called **torque**.

Just as there are various ways of applying a force, so too are there different types of strength. Cast iron for instance has high compressive strength but very low tensile strength. The famous Iron Bridge, built in 1779 over the Severn in Shropshire, was the first large cast iron structure. It was essential in this structure to keep the forces in compression which is why it was built as an arch. In contrast, the Menai suspension bridge, designed and built in 1818 by Telford, used wrought iron (fairly pure iron) in tension. The modern Severn bridge in the County of Avon also uses steel tension cables but modern high tensile steels allow the structure to be much lighter.

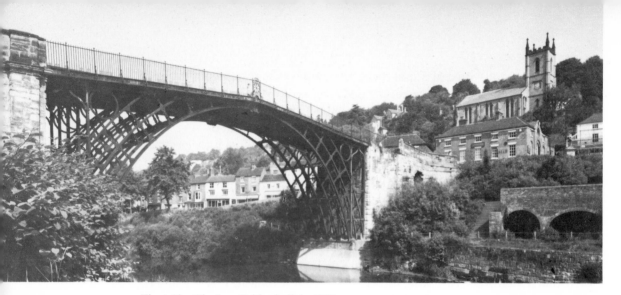

Fig. 1.12   The Iron Bridge built in 1779

Fig. 1.13   The Severn Suspension Bridge completed in 1966

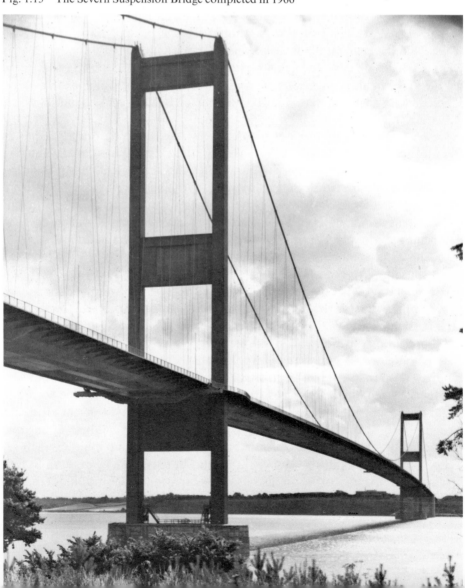

Hardness is the ability to withstand wear, scratching or indentation. You have probably been impressed at the ease with which a skilled man can cut glass. He can of course use a diamond, which is the hardest of all materials, as the cutting edge of the tool, or a tungsten carbide tip which is a much cheaper man-made equivalent.

All cutting tools rely on the blades being harder than the material they have to cut. Scissors, shears, knives, drills and lathe tools are common examples of tools where hardness is essential. Glasspaper, emery cloth and garnet paper are perhaps less obvious cutting tools, but abrasives nevertheless depend upon hardness to be effective.

Hardness is also essential for scribing tools where reliability and long service are of importance. An aircraft flight recorder consists of a diamond stylus scribing lines on a stainless steel tape. The lines permanently record the aircraft performance, data invaluable to investigators of aircraft accidents.

Fig. 1.14   A flight recorder recovered from the wreckage of an aeroplane

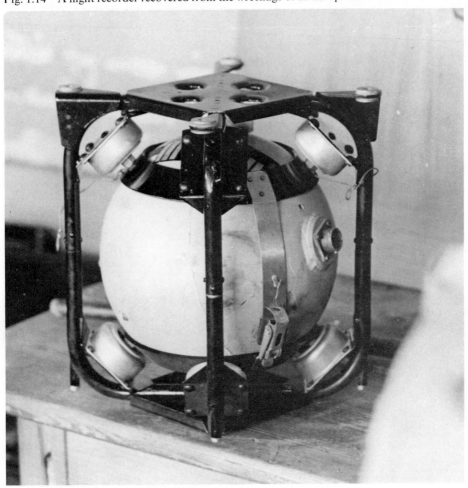

2 Atomic Structure and Crystallisation

■ Elements and Compounds

When certain substances are heated they decompose. Such substances are called **compounds**. A compound is any material which can be broken down into simpler chemical substances.

The compound limestone (or chalk) for instance is often heated at quarries in large furnaces or retorts to yield the very important material quicklime which is used to make mortar and cement. The gas carbon dioxide is the other chemical formed.

Fig. 2.1   Breaking down limestone by heat into quicklime for cement and carbon dioxide

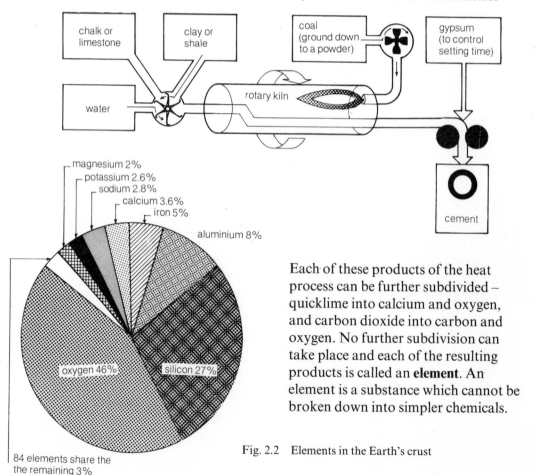

Each of these products of the heat process can be further subdivided – quicklime into calcium and oxygen, and carbon dioxide into carbon and oxygen. No further subdivision can take place and each of the resulting products is called an **element**. An element is a substance which cannot be broken down into simpler chemicals.

Fig. 2.2   Elements in the Earth's crust

84 elements share the the remaining 3% of the Earth's crust

22

If all the chemicals in the Earth's crust, the sea and the atmosphere were broken down into their elements in a similar way to the limestone, we would find that some elements were far more common than others (Fig. 2.2).

The earlier known elements were the metals found in, or easily obtained from, the Earth, i.e. copper, tin, gold, silver, lead and iron. We now know that there are 92 naturally occurring elements and that everything in the world is made up from chemicals containing these elements.

■ Atoms and Molecules

An **atom** of an element is the smallest part into which that element can be chemically divided.

The particles of a compound consist of two or more different atoms joined together. For instance the gas carbon dioxide, formed during the production of quicklime, consists of one atom of carbon joined to two atoms of oxygen. This arrangement is called a **molecule**.

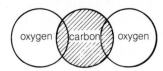

Fig. 2.3   A molecule of carbon dioxide

A molecule is the smallest particle of a compound or an element which will show the properties of the material. One atom will always combine with another in order to form a molecule.

■ Inside Different Atoms

Although there are 92 different kinds of atom, one for each element, each atom has the same basic structure. The main difference is in their size and weight.

Every atom is rather like a miniature solar system. There is a very dense, tiny centre called a **nucleus** which has a positive electric charge. It is from this part of the atom that **nuclear energy** comes. Orbiting around the nucleus, rather like planets around the sun, are very light particles with a negative electric charge known as **electrons**. These are very important and largely determine how an element behaves physically and chemically.

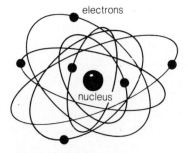

Fig. 2.4   The atom

In some elements some of these electrons in the outermost orbit, or shell, are very loose and can easily be detached from the atom. These elements are metals. In others, the non-metals, they are tightly bound to the nucleus. It is this which makes metals in general good conductors and makes non-metals insulators.

All molecules or atoms are attracted to one another by the electrical forces they set up, some more strongly than others. These electrical forces of attraction, like those between the positively charged nucleus and negatively charged electrons, hold materials together.

■ Ionic Bonding

In industry, when an object has to be coated with an expensive metal such as chromium or copper, one of the best methods of doing this is by using a process known as **electroplating**. This uses a direct current flowing through a liquid (known as an **electrolyte**) to deposit the metal on to the negative terminal of the bath. The chemical name for this is **electrolysis**.

Electrolysis, as well as being a very useful technological process (it is used for refining metals as well as electroplating), can tell us a lot about the forces of attraction holding some materials together.

If, for instance, some copper chloride (a blue crystalline solid) is dissolved in water, electricity can be made to pass through it with the aid of a small 6 V battery and a pair of graphite terminals. After a short time, the **cathode** connected to the negative terminal of the battery will become coated with a pink-coloured metal (copper) while a gas is given off at the positive terminal, the **anode**. This gas is chlorine and is poisonous in concentrated doses.

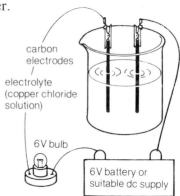

carbon electrodes

electrolyte (copper chloride solution)

6V bulb

6V battery or suitable dc supply

Fig. 2.5   Electrolysis of copper chloride solution

The electric current is separating the molecules of copper chloride into atoms of copper and chlorine. It would seem that because the copper is being attracted to the negative terminal, it must itself be positively charged in the solution (like charges repel, unlike charges attract). Chlorine, by a similar argument, is obviously negatively charged.

In the solid crystal of copper chloride, it is the opposing charges of copper and chlorine that hold the crystal together. Another material held together by similar forces is common salt (sodium chloride). Figure 2.6 shows how the electrical forces between the positively and negatively charged atoms hold the material together to form a **cubic crystal lattice**. When millions of these

Fig. 2.6   Ionic bonding

● positive sodium ions

○ negative sodium ions

'atoms' come together, they form little cubes of salt that can be seen quite clearly under a normal microscope.

An atom with an electrical charge is known as an **ion** and thus the forces attracting the positive and negative ions are known as **ionic bonds**.

☐ Covalent Bonding

Many materials of technological importance, both liquid and solid, are held together by a different type of force called **covalent bonding**. Among the types of materials that fall into this group are many of the rocks and sands widely mined and quarried in this country as the basis of the construction industry. Many of the organic products available directly or indirectly from the natural world are also classified in this way. An organic material is one which is derived from something that is, or has been. alive. Oils and wood are good examples.

This type of bonding is more complex structurally than ionic bonding. It consists of two types of atoms which overlap one another in such a way that they share some of their electrons to make their outer orbits complete. The atoms themselves, however, are not electrically charged and so the material is not affected by electricity. In fact all covalently bonded materials are electrical insulators. Figure 2.7 shows a water molecule, with the two hydrogen atoms sharing two of the oxygen's outer orbit electrons to make their own orbits appear complete. Oil is a typical example and is composed of hydrogen and carbon atoms. It is referred to as a **hydrocarbon**.

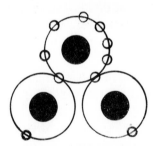

Fig. 2.7   Covalent bonding

☐ Metallic Bonding

Although metals do vary in some properties such as their density and strength, they have much in common with each other. In general they are shiny solids, good conductors of heat and electricity, in addition to numerous other important physical properties. The reason for these similarities is that the atoms of metals are joined together by similar forces, called **metallic bonding**.

Each metal atom has usually one or two electrons attached to it that are very loose and which orbit in the outer electron shell. In the metal crystal these electrons are free to move from one part of the crystal to another and to latch on to any atom for a short time before moving on again.

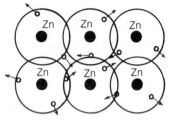

o→ free electrons

Fig. 2.8   Metallic bonding

The presence of free electrons explains the electrical conductivity of metals. Applying a voltage to the conductor will 'excite' the atoms causing an increased but organised movement of the free electrons. The movement of electrons becomes an electric current as they drift round the circuit.

A heat source causes similar agitation (without the organisation) and the excited electrons communicate their agitation to others, thus allowing heat to be conducted through the material.

■ Crystallisation

To some people the word 'crystal' generally suggests either cut glass or crystals such as copper sulphate grown in a chemistry laboratory. However, there are very many other 'crystalline' materials to be found.

A **crystal** is simply a substance with an organised structure. The atoms or molecules of the material are joined together to form definite regular patterns. Look closely at a galvanised (zinc coated) steel dustbin and you will clearly see that the zinc is made of crystalline areas between one and two centimetres in length. All metals are crystalline although it is not always easy to see this feature without a microscope.

Many rocks formed as the Earth cooled millions of years ago are crystalline too. Quartz, calcite, ruby and fluorspar are good examples and are very beautiful to look at.

However, many materials that are not so obviously crystalline are still made up of crystals. Materials like the graphite in your pencil lead, the nylon from which some of your clothes are made, or the polypropylene from which many moulded plastic chairs are manufactured are examples of crystalline materials. Others which you may think of as crystals such as crystal glass, for instance, are **amorphous**. An amorphous material is one in which the atoms or molecules are distributed in a jumbled or haphazard way.

A simple comparison may help us here. Many of you will have been to a football or rugby match at a large stadium. Part of the ground is terraced and people stand in this area in a haphazard fashion rather like molecules in an amorphous substance. In the grandstand, however, people sit in seats laid out in rows and so they are organised rather like the atoms or molecules in a crystal.

As a material such as molten metal cools slowly from the liquid state, the atoms bond themselves together permanently, often forming long thin fernlike crystals known as **dendrites**. Gradually these dendrites grow together to form a crystalline solid. The crystals have packed themselves together like pieces in a jigsaw puzzle. The frost on a window causes the same phenomenon as the droplets of water crystallise into ice.

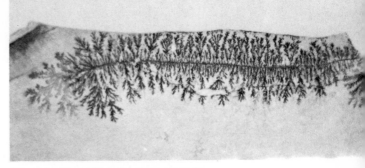

Fig. 2.9   Dendrites of manganese oxide formed within layers of limestone

In metals, these crystals are often so small that they can only be seen after the metal has been polished flat and then **etched** with a weak chemical solution. This procedure reveals a honeycomb of boundaries dividing the metal into areas called **grains**.

Observing the crystalline structure of metal through a microscope is an experience similar to looking at an image in a kaleidoscope. The light is scattered off the crystal faces which are inclined at very many different angles. Each grain is a single crystal and metal consists of many such grains joined together along common boundaries.

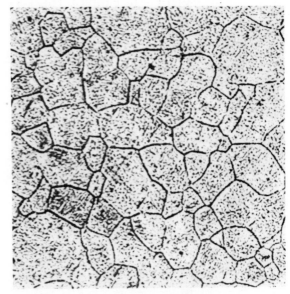

Fig. 2.10   Grain boundaries in iron (magnification × 50)

Fig. 2.11   Grain boundaries in brass (magnification × 500)

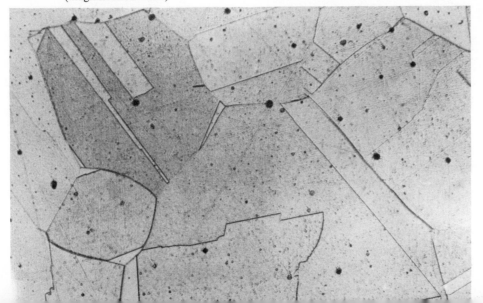

☐ Crystal Shapes

We can get some idea of how the
molecules or atoms are joined together
in some crystals by looking at their
shape. For instance, grains of salt
appear as tiny cubes when viewed
through a hand lens. The sodium and
chlorine ions of salt crystals are
arranged to form the cubic pattern
shown in Fig. 2.12

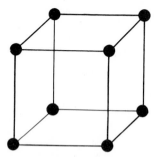

Fig. 2.12   The simple cubic pattern
of salt crystals

The pattern into which the atoms form is known as a **crystal lattice**. To save
showing the whole of the crystal lattice in order to describe a crystal pattern, it
is often more convenient to show only the smallest part of it which will reveal
the pattern in its entirety. This is known as the **unit cell** of the crystal lattice.
Some of these unit cells are shown in Figs. 2.13 to 2.15.

We will now look at the most common ways in which the molecules in a
substance can arrange themselves. One crystal shape in metals is known as the
close-packed hexagonal (cph) structure. This is the most densely packed of the
molecular structures as each layer of atoms sits displaced by half a molecular
diameter in each direction, so that each atom sits in the 'cup' between the atoms
in the layer below. Zinc and magnesium are examples of metals displaying this
crystal structure.

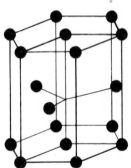

Fig. 2.13   (a) Close-packed hexagonal crystalline structure

(b) Stages in building a cph model

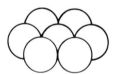
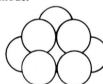
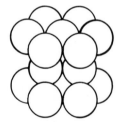

Another common crystal form is the **body-centred cubic** (bcc) structure. In this
crystal the atoms arrange themselves into a cubic structure with an extra atom
sitting in the centre of each cube. Chromium, molybdenum, tungsten, and iron
at room temperature have this structure.

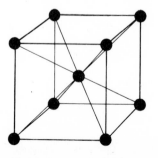

Fig. 2.14   (a) Body-centred cubic crystalline structure

(b) A bcc model

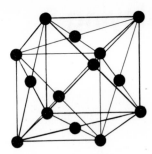 Fig. 2.15 (a) Face-centred cubic crystalline structure

(b) Stages in building an fcc model

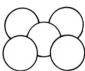 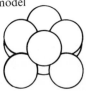 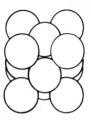

A **face-centred cubic** (fcc) structure is another modification. As the name suggests, each face of the cube has an additional atom sitting in its centre. Iron at high temperatures, copper, silver, gold, aluminium, nickel and lead have this structure.

3 The Extraction and Alloying of Metals

■ Extraction

Metals are rarely found in their pure state and are generally chemically combined with other substances, in particular oxygen and sulphur. In order to obtain the metals in their useful form, they have to be extracted from the ore by a series of processes.

Mining or **quarrying** involves extracting the ore mixed with earth, clay or rocks. It would be uneconomical to transport large quantities of waste material from the mine head to the smelter so the ore is first of all **crushed** so that it can be **concentrated** to remove much of the waste.

Metallic ores
↓
Mining or quarrying
↓
Crushing
↓
Concentrating
↓
Roasting
↙   ↘
Smelting   Electrolysis
↘   ↙
Metal
↓
Refining

Fig. 3.1   Iron ore being unloaded at an ore terminal

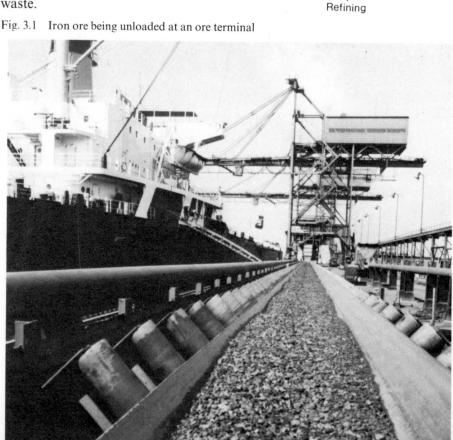

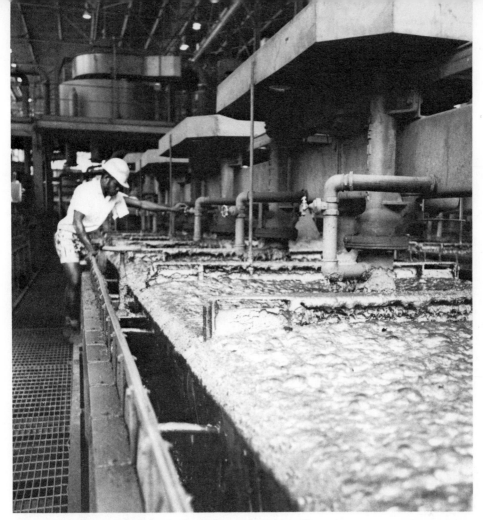

Fig. 3.2   Concentrate frothing to the surface in flotation cells

One modern technique of concentration is by **froth flotation** where violent air agitation suspends the crushed ore in water to which frothing agents have been added. By careful control of the frothing agents, the required metallic ores are picked up in the bubbles while the waste material sinks. The froth containing the ore is skimmed off. This technique is so effective in separating different ores that it is one of the factors which made it again possible to extract metals on a profitable basis from some Cornish mines which had been previously forced to close.

Having mined and then concentrated the ore, the next stage of the extraction process is **roasting**. This causes the ore to change chemically into an oxide of the metal.

The final stage is to break the chemical bond between the metal and the oxygen in the ore. This process is called **reduction** and varies in certain details depending on the metal and the ease with which the chemical bond can be broken.

■ Reduction

The different atomic structure of each element determines the ease with which it will form compounds. The elements which are more reactive take part in chemical reactions more readily. We can list these in order of reactivity.

More reactive	Magnesium
	Aluminium
	Carbon
	Zinc
	Iron
	Tin
	Lead
Less reactive	Copper

The order of reactivity determines the process of reduction that is used. Each material can be reduced by heating it with any one of the more reactive metals that is above it. Consider the reduction of lead oxide with carbon. Carbon is chemically more reactive than lead (see list), and the carbon will take the oxygen from the lead oxide to produce metallic lead.

Carbon is a useful chemical in the reduction process because it is cheap and can be used to extract those metals below it in the order of reactivity. The carbon used is in the form of coke.

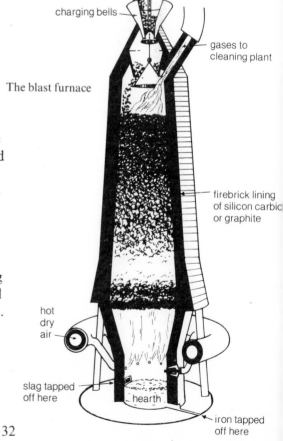

Fig. 3.3   The blast furnace

charging bells

gases to cleaning plant

firebrick lining of silicon carbic or graphite

hot dry air

slag tapped off here

hearth

iron tapped off here

■ The Production of Iron

When smelting iron, the ore and coke are fed into a blast furnace and heated to 1600°C. One other important addition is limestone which combines with the impurities to form a molten slag which floats on the heavier iron. The iron and slag are tapped off separately and the iron is poured into large containers. The iron is called pig iron and is still too impure for general use and will have to be further refined. The pig iron is converted into steel by transferring ladles of molten metal to convertor furnaces which reduce the impurities and control the carbon content.

32

■ The Production of Aluminium

For the metals above carbon on the list, no cheap chemical is available for reduction. The extraction of aluminium relies on passing an electric current through the molten aluminium oxide to break the chemical bond.

Aluminium ore (bauxite) is obtained by open cast mining and concentrated by dissolving in hot caustic soda to remove impurities. After dissolving the aluminium oxide in caustic soda it forms sodium aluminate. Carbon dioxide is passed through and precipitates aluminium hydroxide. The aluminium hydroxide is then roasted to produce aluminium oxide once more but in a purified state.

When the oxide is mixed with a mineral called **cryolite** its melting point is lowered to 1000°C. By passing a high electric current through it, the aluminium oxide is split into aluminium, which is collected at the base of the electric cell, and oxygen which is released as a gas. This electrolytic process results in a very pure aluminium that needs no further refining.

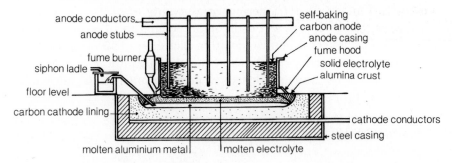

Fig. 3.4   The electrolytic reduction cell

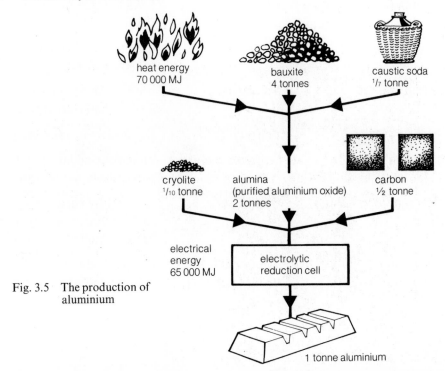

Fig. 3.5   The production of aluminium

The graph (Fig. 3.6) compares the total energy input per tonne for steel and aluminium. The enormous energy input for aluminium is explained by the electrical energy needed to break the aluminium oxide bond.

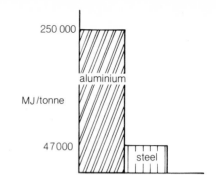

Fig. 3.6   The total energy input per tonne for steel and aluminium

◼ Alloying

Metals are rarely used in their pure state because they are often too soft and ductile. Instead, they are often alloyed to increase strength or hardness. However, many other properties will be altered either intentionally or otherwise, e.g. colour, electrical or thermal conductivity.

The following list gives some of the more common alloys and their applications. This list is very general and within each class of alloy there will be very many different proportions of the same metals. In addition, only the two major components of the alloy are listed, whereas in practice the alloy may often contain small proportions of other metals.

COMMON ALLOYS AND THEIR APPLICATIONS

Components	Alloy	Uses
Copper and zinc	Brass	Locks, watch mechanisms, electrical fittings.
Copper and tin	Bronze	Castings, bells, statues, hard solder, bearings.
Lead and tin	Solder	Many different proportions give solders with different uses.
Tin and lead	Pewter	Decorative metalwork.
Tin and antimony	Babbitt's metal	Plain bearing liners particularly for aircraft.
Zinc and aluminium	'Mazak'	Diecastings such as carburettors, pumps, car door handles, pulleys.
Lead and antimony	Type metal, white metal	Printers' type, plain bearings for cars, radiation protection shields, battery plates.

34

Nickel and chromium	Nichrome, nimonic	Resistance wires, jet engines.
Copper and nickel	Monel, cupro-nickel, nickel silver	Mine sweeper hulls, propeller shafts, coins (50p, 10p).
Magnesium and aluminium	'Magnox'	Atomic reactor fuel cans, engine blocks, aircraft castings, cameras, textile machinery.
Steel and chromium	Stainless steel	Sinks, cutlery, medical uses where sterile conditions are important.

The most common reason for alloying is to increase strength. Figure 3.7 shows how copper is strengthened by adding aluminium. The addition of 7% aluminium to copper produces an alloy nearly twice as strong as pure copper. With 10% aluminium content the alloy approaches three times the strength of pure copper. The alloy, known as aluminium bronze, is as strong as mild steel, very tough, and is a valuable engineering material.

Fig. 3.7   The effect of aluminium on the strength of copper aluminium alloys

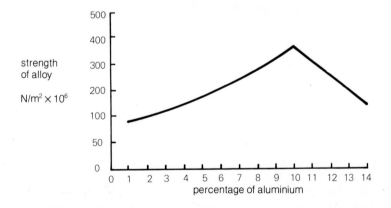

Further increases in the aluminium content lead to a steady reduction in the strength of the alloy, but at the other end of this copper-aluminium series, alloys rich in aluminium and containing up to 12% copper are again useful. The high strength of aluminium bronze is not reached but nevertheless these alloys are considerably stronger than pure aluminium with only a marginal increase in weight.

A similar pattern emerges if you compare the strength versus the carbon content in steel (Fig. 3.8). Notice the very small quantities of carbon that are

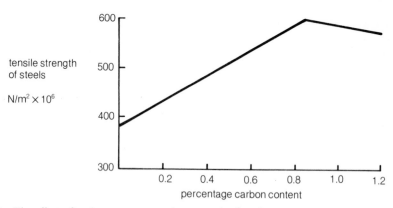

Fig. 3.8   The effect of carbon content on the strength of steels

needed to produce dramatic increases in strength. Once again you will notice that tensile strength decreases after a certain stage.

Type of iron/steel	Approximate carbon content
Mild steel	up to 0.25%
Medium carbon steel	0.25–0.45%
High carbon steel	0.45–1.5%
Cast iron	2.5 –4.5%

Hardness is another property affected by alloying. Small amounts of an 'impurity' element will interfere with the regularity of the slip planes in a metal and it will become harder. For example, 0.5% of magnesium is sufficient to harden aluminium.

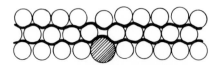

Fig. 3.9   Simplified illustration of the effect of an 'impure' atom on slip planes

■ The Melting Point of Alloys

In almost all cases, the melting point of a metal is lowered by alloying it with another. This is not an unnatural occurrence if you compare it to what happens when salt is put down on an icy road. In this case, the mixture of salt and water has a lower freezing point than that of pure water. The same effect is to be found in metallurgy.

By a careful choice of constituents, it is possible to make alloys with unusually low melting points. An alloy of four or five metals can be mixed so that the lowest melting point possible is obtained. A fusible alloy, known as Wood's metal, has a composition by weight of four parts bismuth, two parts lead, one part tin and one part cadmium. Its melting point is about 70°C, i.e., less than the boiling point of water. Practical jokers can amuse themselves with a teaspoon made of Wood's metal which will melt when used to stir a hot cup of tea.

A technological use for such low melting point alloys is in automatic fire sprinkler systems. Each jet is sealed with a piece of fusible alloy which melts and releases water in the event of an outbreak of fire.

The alloying of tin and lead to make solder is another good example where the lower melting point of the alloy has important uses. Lead melts at 327°C and tin at 232°C. If lead is added to molten tin, the melting point of the alloy is always lower than the melting points of lead or tin.

☐ The Melting of Tin/Lead Alloys

The graph shows the melting characteristics of tin/lead alloys. Consider the alloy of 90% tin and 10% lead. On cooling, the mixture reaches a temperature of 217°C before it begins to solidify. As the alloy cools further, it gradually changes from a fluid state, through a stage like paste and gradually becomes thicker. Finally, at a temperature of 183°C, the whole alloy has become completely solid.

Fig. 3.10   The melting characteristics of tin/lead alloys

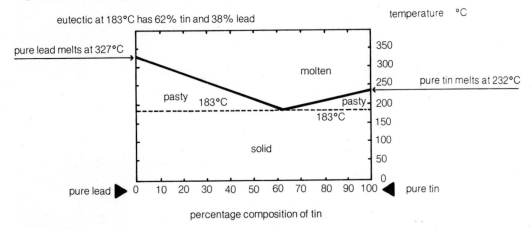

A plumber makes use of a long 'pasty' stage in the solidification to give him time to make a 'wiped joint'. Plumber's solder has 70% lead and 30% tin.

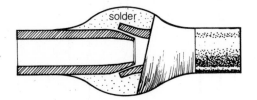

Fig. 3.11   A 'wiped joint'

37

Modern lead-sheathed telecommunication cables are widely used by the Post Office. The joining of sections of these cables still requires the properties of a solder that will make a joint similar to the plumber's 'wiped joint'. Such solders are also used in car body filling, particularly in the roof to gutter joints.

Solders rich in lead and containing very little tin are used for soldering parts of car radiators where the temperatures require that the solder has an even higher melting point.

Look at Fig. 3.10 again. With 80% tin, the alloy starts solidifying at 203°C and finishes at 183°C. Note the recurrence of this latter temperature.

One particular alloy, containing 62% tin and 38% lead, melts and solidifies entirely at 183°C. Obviously this temperature of 183°C and the 62/38 per cent composition are important in the tin/lead alloy system. Similar effects occur in many other alloy systems; the special composition of each series which has the lowest freezing point and which entirely freezes at that temperature is known as the **eutectic** alloy. The freezing temperature (183°C in the case of the tin/lead alloy) is called the **eutectic temperature**.

This eutectic alloy melts to a free flowing liquid which will penetrate minute openings. It is used for soldering electronic circuits where minimum heat is required because of sensitive components.

4 Cold Working and Heat Treatment

■ Mechanical Cold Working

Most people, at some time or another, have tried to break a piece of metal by bending it backwards and forwards. Before it eventually fractures two noticeable things happen; the metal becomes more and more difficult to bend and gets fairly hot. The metal has been **'work hardened'**.

Many of the manufacturing techniques in metal working rely on the ease with which metal can be shaped through its ductility, and the increased strength that results from work hardening. Virtually all the body panels of a car are work hardened while being formed between very large dies.

The way in which many fastenings such as rivets, screws and bolts are manufactured are examples of cold forming techniques. A modern bolt-making machine feeds a thick wire into a steel die, Stage 1. A second die swells the protruding metal, Stage 2. The head is next trimmed to the finished shape, Stage 3. Finally the workpiece has to be threaded. The thread is formed on the shank by a process known as **thread rolling**. Cold-rolled threads have several advantages over cut threads; the accuracy can be much more closely controlled and the bolt is 13% stronger due to the **plastic flow** in the thread structure. The complex pattern of Phillips recessed head screws as well as other less common screw heads are produced by this process.

Fig. 4.1 Stages in making a bolt

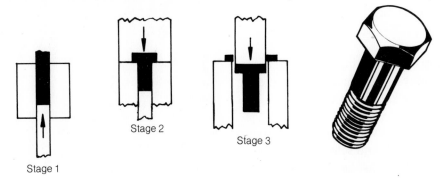

Stage 2

Stage 3

Stage 1

Apart from the increased strength of cold formed products, the process is also attractive because there is very little waste metal (Fig. 4.2).

39

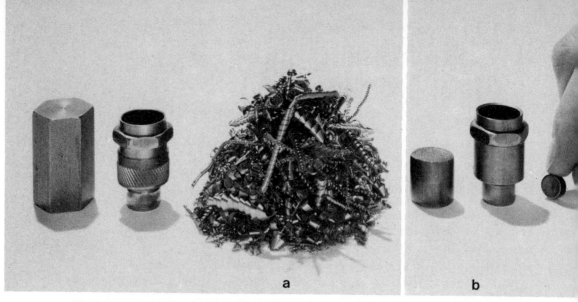

Fig. 4.2 (a) Traditional machined component and waste metal produced
(b) Component re-designed for cold forming, showing the reduction in waste metal and also the saving in raw material

If components are to be shaped by processes such as cold forming, the metal must be ductile.

□ Dislocations

As the process of crystallisation takes place, gaps between the atoms of the crystals interrupt the crystalline order and often produce a line of defects. These defects in metals are known as **dislocations** and help to explain why metals are ductile.

Compare the stretching of a metal to a large display of cans in a supermarket. Perfectly stacked, it is a very stable structure. We can all visualise the catastrophe that will happen if we give in to temptation and select a can from the centre of the display. In a similar but not catastrophic way, vacancies in a crystal lattice promote movement of the atoms when a force is applied.

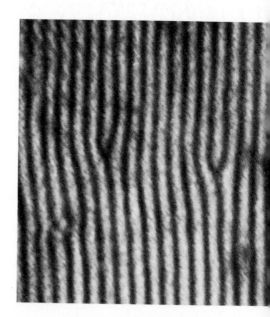

Fig. 4.3 Dislocations in gold film revealed by moiré fringe techniques

Dislocations are doing just this and can be thought of as atoms rolling over

40

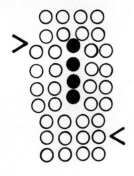 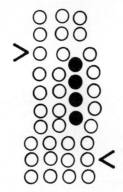 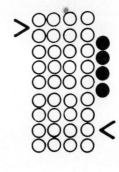

Fig. 4.4   (a) Edge dislocation   (b) Dislocation sheared   (c) Dislocation sheared
                                                   one lattice spacing   out of crystal

each other to make a forward movement. What happens to these dislocations
as they move through a metal? The grain boundaries of the metal form natural
barriers which prevent further movement of the dislocations. The metal then
becomes hard and brittle.

■ **Annealing**

Annealing is the softening process applied to a metal by heating and allowing it
to cool slowly. It is a process which is carried out on a metal that has been work
hardened and on which further work could not be effected without causing it to
fracture. The annealed metal is now in its softest state and has the ductility to
accept further stretching. Annealing can therefore be seen to have the opposite
effect to cold working on the mechanical properties of a metal. The heating
process has to be done at a sufficiently high temperature for the particular
metal so that the atoms will move energetically enough to **recrystallise**. The
process of recrystallisation, however, usually takes place well below the
melting point of the metal.

■ **Surface Hardening**

The purpose of heat treatment is to alter the mechanical properties of a metal.
Annealing aims at making a metal softer or more ductile. Heat treatment aims
to make the metal stronger and harder.

Surface hardening is a process applied to low-carbon steels. By heating the
steel in a carbon-rich material, the carbon can diffuse into the surface of the
steel. A surface treated in this way could now be reheated and quenched in oil
or water to produce a very hard skin. A surface-hardened steel has the
advantage of retaining the toughness of low carbon steel in its core with a
surface hardness that will resist abrasion. Gear wheels are a good example
where such properties are necessary.

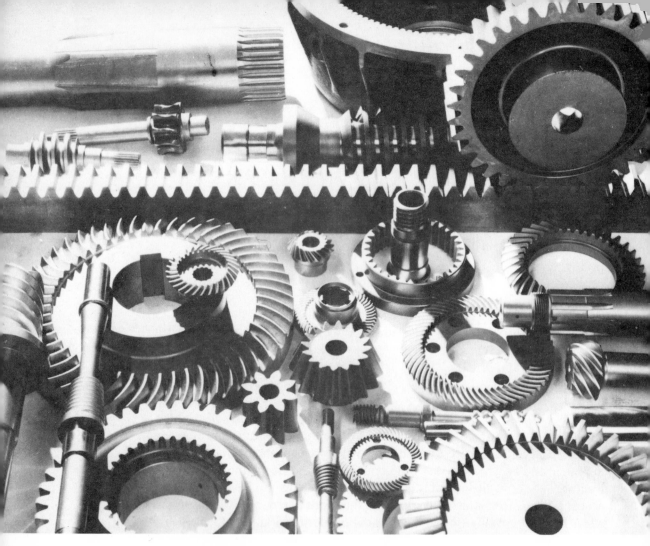

Fig. 4.5   A selection of gear wheels

☐ Hardening and Tempering

To harden high-carbon steel containing 0.8% carbon, it has to be heated above 733°C (cherry-red heat in daylight) and quenched in oil or water. The result is a dramatic increase in hardness and brittleness. This state is often called 'glass hard' because the steel will shatter very easily. Because they break so easily, tools in this condition have little use. More toughness is needed without sacrificing too much hardness, and this is achieved by a second operation known as **tempering**.

The steel is carefully heated to a pre-determined temperature, between 200°C and 300°C, followed by quenching in oil or water. The exact temperature depends upon the purpose of the tool or article. Tools in the lower temperature range have a high degree of hardness, but poor shock resistance, while in the upper range, good shock resistance but less hardness. Coloured oxides of iron, which appear on the steel as it is heated, give an approximate guide to the temperature as shown below.

	°C	Tempering Colour	Article
Decreasing hardness but increasing toughness	290	Blue	Screwdrivers, springs
↑	275	Purple	Axes, chisels, punches
	260	Brown	Lathe centres, plane irons
↓	240	Dark straw	Dies, knives, taps
Increasing hardness	230	Light straw	Lathe tools
and brittleness	220	Yellow	Dividers, scalpels, scrapers, scribers

☐ The Heat Treatment of Aluminium Alloys

Aluminium alloys can also be heat treated in a two-stage process. In the first heat treatment called **solution treatment**, the alloying elements dissolve in the aluminium and quenching keeps them in solid solution. In a solid solution atoms of the unit cell of one element are replaced by atoms of the alloying elements. The solution-treated material is then reheated for the **precipitation treatment** which permits a phase rich in the alloy elements to precipitate, or settle out, under controlled conditions.

This process of precipitation which hardens and strengthens the alloy sometimes occurs unaided over a period of time. In the case of Duralumin, an aluminium alloy containing 4% of copper, the copper atoms migrate from the homogeneous solid solution of copper in aluminium to form copper rich regions. This natural process is called **age hardening**.

Fig. 4.6 (a) Minority atoms in a solid solution   (b) Precipitation hardening collects together the minority atoms to strain the lattice

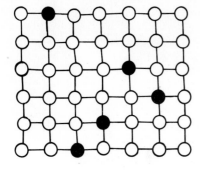
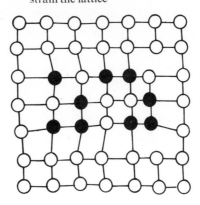

5 Factors Influencing the Application of Metals

■ The Forming of Metals

Once a metal has been extracted from its ore and refined, it is ready to be produced in commercial form. Industry may require the metal in sheet form to be pressed into shape for car bodies or containers, or it may be required in the form of bars, perhaps for reinforcing concrete, or girders for bridges and buildings. Wire is also needed for electrical cable or wire rope. Most metals are rolled or squeezed into these stock shapes at a rolling mill.

Metal from a furnace is now rarely cast into moulds to make ingots, which would require later reheating at the rolling mill. Instead, a method called **continuous casting** delivers red-hot metal in convenient-sized slabs or blooms direct to the rolling mill for immediate shaping. The slabs are rolled into strip or sheet, and the blooms may be reduced in size to square or round stock, or be formed into girders and angles. The rolling mill provides industry with metal in stock form for **fabrication** by cutting, shaping, machining and assembly.

Other shaping processes can often bypass these costly stages of rolling by being formed directly from blooms into near finished products.

Fig. 5.1   Continuous horizontal casting of aluminium billets

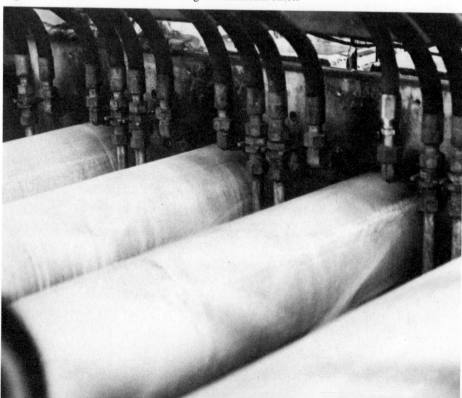

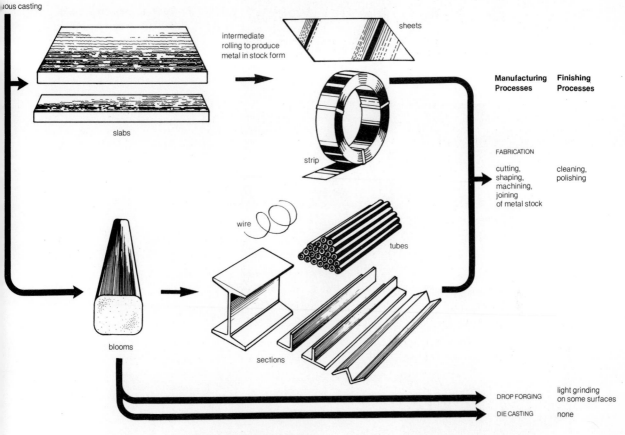

Fig. 5.2   The production of metals in commercial form

■ Casting

Casting is one of the simplest methods of shaping, and involves pouring molten metal into a prepared mould where it solidifies into the shape of the mould. Depending on the size, complexity and material to be used, casting is often more economic than other production methods. It is intended to reduce machining operations to a minimum.

Sand moulding is the traditional way of achieving a complicated casting. A pattern, or copy, of the final article is packed in special moulding sand and then removed to leave a cavity into which the metal is poured. The process is still used for large castings but is being replaced by cleaner and faster techniques such as shell moulding and die casting.

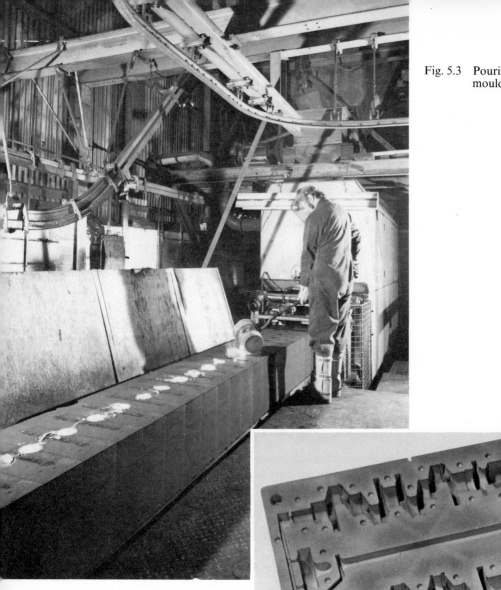

Fig. 5.3 Pouring metal into sand moulds

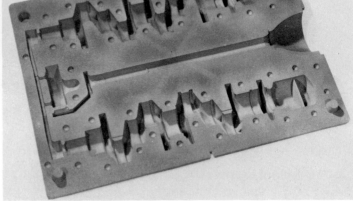

Fig. 5.4 One half of a shell mould

Shell moulding has superseded much of the heavy sand moulds. A steel pattern is sprayed with a resin and is dusted with a thin layer of sand before being baked in an oven. When the steel mould is removed, a thin shell of resin and sand remains into which the metal is poured.

When very large quantities of the same components are needed, it is more economic to make a hollow steel mould and cast metal into it. This process is called **die casting** and components can be made to a very high degree of accuracy. The molten metal is supplied to the mould under high pressure which ensures accuracy and a good quality surface finish. Carburettors and engine blocks are made in this way.

Fig. 5.5   A die casting machine in operation

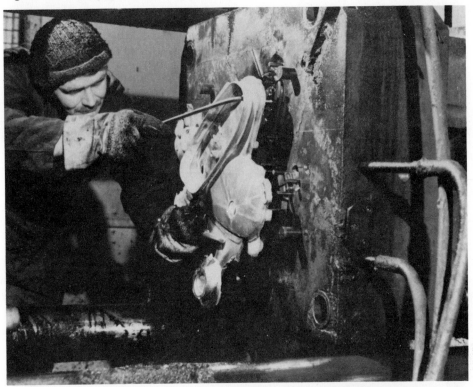

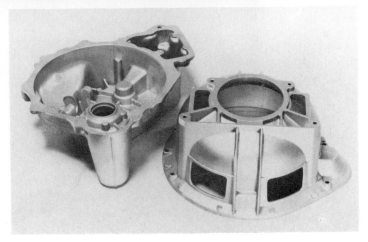

Fig. 5.6   Typical die castings for the
automobile industry

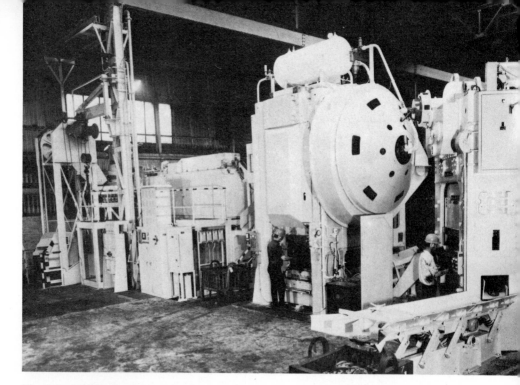

Fig. 5.7 A 2000 t forging press

■ Drop Forging

In this process the hot metal is squeezed between two shaped steel dies. Under the force of the die that is dropped, the metal takes up the internal shape of the dies. Successive dies may be necessary when the component has a complicated shape, e.g. a crankshaft for a piston engine. Only a limited amount of machining may be necessary to finish such a component. Hammer heads and gear blanks are also made by drop forging.

Fig. 5.8 A selection of drop forgings

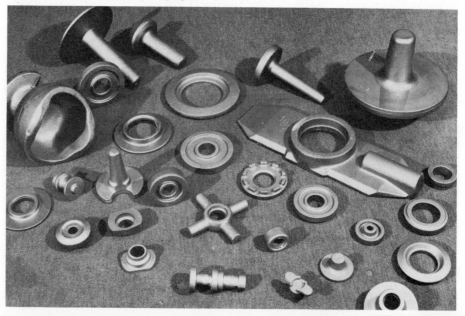

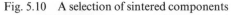

Fig. 5.9   The sintering process

upper punch

powder in die cavity

lower punch

compact

▉ Sintering

By fusing together fine metal particles, the sintering process is capable of producing small intricate components very precisely. The metal powder is compressed at high pressure in a die to form a compact of the required shape.

The compact is removed from the die and sintered by heating it in an atmosphere of hydrogen and carbon monoxide. These gases reduce the oxide skin of the metal particles so that they become welded together at a temperature significantly below the melting point of the alloy.

In order to offset the high costs of the press tools, sintering is mainly used for components required in large quantities.

Fig. 5.10   A selection of sintered components

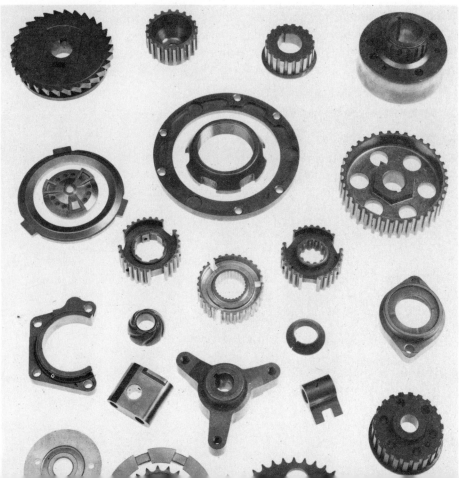

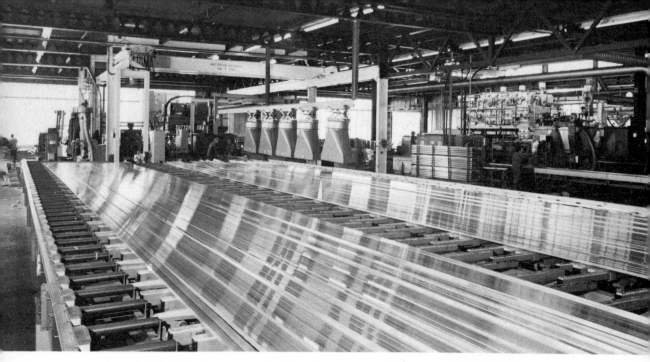

Fig. 5.11   The production of aluminium extrusions from a 1600 t hydraulic press

■ Extrusion

This process is similar to squeezing toothpaste from a tube. The solid metal is forced at a high temperature through a specially shaped die, then cooled and cut. Long lengths of highly complex sections can be produced in this way.

Fig. 5.12   Some typical aluminium extrusions

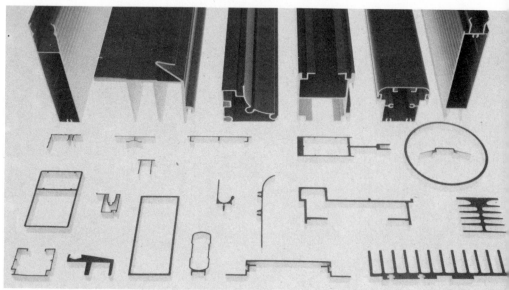

■ Wire Drawing

When the metal is pulled through a die, the process is known as drawing. Wire is made by drawing the metal through several dies with successively smaller apertures.

■ The Tensile Test

A tensile force can be applied to determine the ultimate tensile strength or breaking point of a material. Though we rarely use materials to their breaking point, the list below serves as a useful guide to their tensile strength.

Material	Tensile Strength MN/m²
High tensile steel	1550
Titanium	1400
Mild steel	500
Aluminium alloys	140–600
Magnesium	300
Cast iron	230
Copper	140

$(1 \text{ MN/m}^2 = 1\,000\,000 \text{ N/m}^2 \text{ or } 1 \times 10^6 \text{ N/m}^2.)$

Titanium, for instance, has ten times the tensile strength of copper. To express this in another way, a piece of copper would need a cross-sectional area ten times greater than that of titanium to resist the same tensile load.

A **tensometer** or tensile testing machine (Fig. 5.13) is designed to apply a controlled tensile force. The samples have a reduced centre portion so that the

Fig. 5.13   A simple tensile testing machine

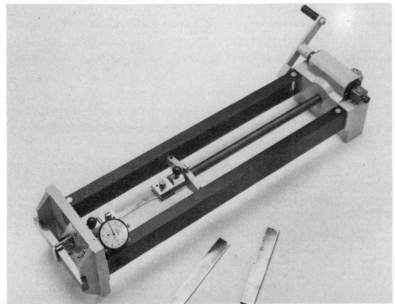

position of the break can be prescribed for observation. The tensile testing machine stretches the material at a constant rate and measures the force needed to do this. The two readings of extension and force can be plotted as a graph to show the performance of the material in terms of its tensile strength.

Fig. 5.14   Force and extension

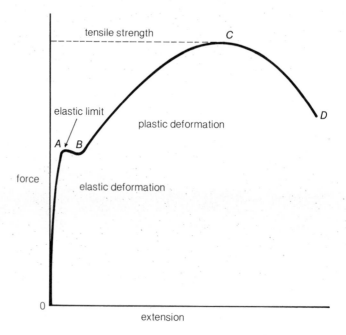

Look at Fig. 5.14. Between *O* and *A* the material is **elastic** and behaves like a spring; it would return to its original length if the load were removed. It obeys Hook's law, i.e. the extension is proportional to the applied force.

Between *A* and *B* the limit of proportionality is reached and the force decreases as **plastic deformation** begins. This phenomenon is known as **yielding**.

Between *B* and *C* the material is deforming plastically. This region of plastic flow is that used in the cold forming processes mentioned previously. At *C* the **ultimate tensile strength** of the specimen is reached, which represents the highest force the material is able to support prior to fracture.

Between *C* and *D* the cross-sectional area of the sample decreases. Before this stage is reached, annealing of cold worked metal would be necessary to prevent fracture during the manufacturing process. Fracture occurs at *D*.

☐ Calculations of Stress, Strain and Young's Modulus

In the next graph (Fig. 5.16) we will compare stress and **strain** rather than force and extension as we did in Fig. 5.14.

52

The stress in a material is the relationship between the applied load and the cross-sectional area of a specimen of the material.

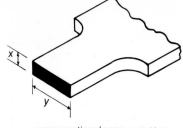

$$\text{Stress} = \frac{\text{load (N)}}{\text{cross-sectional area (m}^2)}.$$

cross-sectional area = $x \times y$

Fig. 5.15   Cross-sectional area

Its unit is N/m^2 (kN/m^2 or MN/m^2). It is usually a very large number.

The strain in a material, often called **fractional strain**, is the relationship between the change in length and the original length of the specimen.

$$\text{Strain} = \frac{\text{change in length}}{\text{original length}}.$$

It has no units. It is usually a very small number, hence the term fractional strain.

Fig. 5.16   Stress and strain

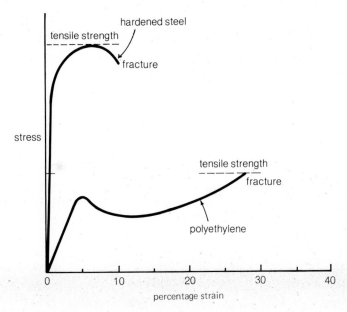

If we wish to indicate the properties of a material in terms of its strength, we use Young's modulus of elasticity. Young discovered that stress is proportional to strain up to the elastic limit (Point A in Fig. 5.14) and this allowed him to make the statement that stress/strain equals a constant. He called his constant a modulus and gave it the symbol E for elasticity,

$$\text{i.e. } \frac{\text{stress}}{\text{strain}} = E.$$

53

$$\text{Since } \frac{\text{stress (N/m}^2)}{\text{strain (number)}} = E,$$

the modulus is stated in N/m^2 and is usually a very large number indeed. In fact the higher the value of E, the greater the strength of the material concerned. Because of its relationship with strain, Young's modulus also indicates the stiffness of a material.

Example

A flat metal stay 500 mm long with a cross section 40 mm $\times$ 50 mm extends 1 mm under a tensile load of 292×10^3 newtons. Calculate (a) the stress in the plate, (b) the strain, (c) Young's modulus for the material.

Cross-sectional area $= 40 \times 10^{-3}$ m $\times 50 \times 10^{-3}$ m $= 2 \times 10^{-3}$ m^2.

(a) Stress $= \dfrac{\text{load}}{\text{cross-sectional area}} = \dfrac{292 \times 10^3}{2 \times 10^{-3}} = 146 \times 10^6$ N/m^2.

(b) Strain $= \dfrac{1 \times 10^{-3}}{0.5} = 2 \times 10^{-3}$.

(c) Young's modulus $= \dfrac{\text{stress}}{\text{strain}} = \dfrac{146 \times 10^6}{2 \times 10^{-3}} = 73 \times 10^9$ N/m^2.

The table gives Young's modulus and tensile strengths for a range of materials.

	Young's Modulus MN/m^2	*Tensile Strength* MN/m^2
High tensile steel	210 000	1550
Mild steel	200 000	500
Carbon fibre composite	200 000	350–1050
Titanium	120 000	700–1400
Graphite	100 000	2000
Copper	96 000	140
Aluminium alloys	73 000	140–600
Glass	70 000	160
Magnesium alloys	42 000	200–300
Brick	21 000	5.5
Concrete	15 000	4.1
Spruce	13 000	10
Polystyrene	3 400	48
Nylon	2 400	60
Polythene	700	20–30
Acrylic	300	60

■ The Hardness Test

There are many instances where hardness is important. If you want to cut something your cutting tool must obviously be harder than the object you wish to cut. Knives, lathe tools, drills, scissors and files are examples of common cutting tools. Abrasives such as carborundum grit, ground glass, garnet and diamond are also used as cutting materials.

One of the drawbacks of a tensile test is that it destroys the material. It has already been mentioned that as materials get stronger they also get harder. With certain metals hardness is directly related to tensile strength. A hardness test is often used for quality control of heat-treated products.

The metal to be tested is placed under a loaded indentor (see Fig. 5.17) for a fixed time. The diameter of the indentation in the metal gives the basis for calculating the area of the dent. The material is given a hardness number which allows it to be compared with others.

Fig. 5.17   A simple hardness tester

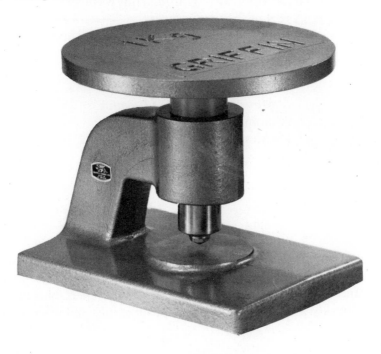

■ Resistance to Corrosion

When iron or steel corrodes we say that it 'rusts'. Rust is the term given to a form of iron oxide. It is unsightly and severely weakens the mechanical properties of steel. We do not say that copper rusts since it is chemically impossible for copper to develop into an iron oxide, but it does tarnish and will corrode if not treated properly. Verdigris, the vivid green stains of tarnishing copper, is a copper carbonate. Corrosion is the general term given to the way in which metals deteriorate.

Paint is probably the most common of all the methods of preventing corrosion, but it takes a lot of surface preparation and care to apply it properly. Even then, the weather and pollution are more than capable of ruining this fragile barrier to corrosion. Some articles cannot be painted, especially where surfaces have to be sterilised or where the paint would get easily damaged, and so other methods must be used such as zinc and cadmium plating.

Tin cans, which are made from a sheet of steel covered by a very thin layer of tin, are the most familiar of all metallic containers. Tin is a relatively expensive metal but it protects the steel without being toxic to food.

It is easy to find other examples of corrosion. Examine a bicycle, car or any other metal object exposed to the weather and you will realise that corrosion is a major problem.

Corrosion is the cause of considerable waste of the world's diminishing mineral resources. To the loss incurred through this waste of materials must be added the high energy cost of their replacement.

The list below gives an indication of the necessary energy input for extracting a range of raw materials.

Material	Total Energy (MJ/tonne)
Aluminium	250 000
Plastics	54 000
Zinc	50 000
Lead	50 000
Iron and steel	47 000
Copper	43 200
Cement	7 250

Although corrosion can take place in the presence of dry gases, many more common cases are caused by the oxidisation of metal in moist air. Electrochemical processes can accelerate corrosion. When ionically bonded chemicals, e.g. salt, are dissolved in water, positive ions and negative ions are liberated.

$$NaCl \xrightarrow{} Na^+ + Cl^-$$
solid salt → salt ions in water

These ions, together with the positive hydrogen ions (H^+) and negative hydroxyl ions (OH^-) of water, are available for conducting electricity through a solution. This generation of electricity during corrosion produces what is called a **corrosion cell**.

The most common useful application of a corrosion cell is a dry cell battery. The electricity flows at the expense of the corroding zinc casing.

Any metal is capable of becoming a corrosion cell due to small differences in composition within the metal itself. Work hardened areas of metal are particularly prone to corrosion.

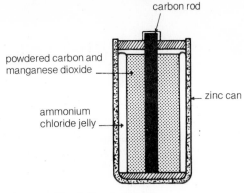

carbon rod

powdered carbon and manganese dioxide

zinc can

ammonium chloride jelly

Fig. 5.18   A dry cell

☐ Bimetallic Corrosion (Galvanic Corrosion)

Whenever two metals are in contact in the presence of moisture, a corrosion cell will be set up between them. It is important to know which metals will corrode more readily and this will depend on their particular environment. Perhaps the most common corrosion environment is sea water. The **Galvanic series** predicts which metals will corrode more readily in this particular environment.

Galvanic Series in Sea Water

Magnesium alloys
Zinc
Aluminium alloys
Mild steel
Stainless steel, 18-8 active
Lead
Tin
Copper
Bronze
Monel
Nickel
Stainless steel, 18-8 passive
Silver
Titanium   ↓
Gold   *Increasingly*
Platinum   *cathodic*
                                         (protected)

The list is a more comprehensive version of the order of reactivity of metals presented earlier. In a corrosion cell the electrons originate from the chemical reactions at the anode. The anode will be the more reactive of the two metals in the cell. It is called the anode because it would be necessary to join the positive terminal of a battery to the anode to reinforce the same current flow. The further apart that metals are in the list, the greater is the electrical activity between them. The metal which forms the cathode in such a corrosion cell has greater protection.

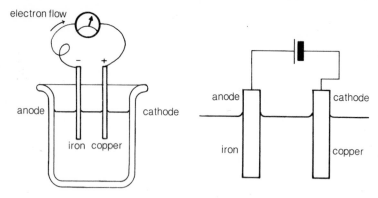

Fig. 5.19   A corrosion cell

Consider a copper plate submerged in sea water and fastened by steel screws. Since copper is lower in the list, the steel screws will corrode. This can be avoided by clamping a piece of aluminium or zinc to the plate. Now the corrosion changes in favour of the aluminium or zinc which is more reactive than steel. The aluminium or zinc is called a **sacrificial anode** since it is being sacrificed in favour of the steel screws.

A common example of a sacrificial anode is a galvanised dustbin. The sheet steel is dipped into hot zinc, and the zinc corrodes instead of the steel at damaged areas, such as scratches which expose the steel. Eventually the zinc will become too corroded and the steel will start to rust.

■ Methods of Preventing Corrosion

1   **Paint**
    The purpose of most paints is to provide a waterproof barrier to prevent corrosion, but unfortunately this barrier is easily scratched or broken. Once the metal is exposed corrosion can start. Some paints such as those rich in zinc attempt to provide a protection of an anodic nature as well as a waterproof barrier.

2   **Plating.**
    Galvanising is one of the more common plating processes achieved by hot dipping metals. Other types of plating such as **chromium plating** are achieved in an electroplating bath.

3   **Anodising.**
    This is an electrical process applied to aluminium and its alloys. Aluminium forms an extremely protective oxide and this oxide depth is increased in the anodising process, giving the material a hard and durable finish. The oxide layer may also be dyed to make it attractive to look at. Similar coloured layers have been developed in recent years on some stainless steels.

58

4 **Plastic Coating.**
Plastic coated steel is now a common method of preventing corrosion. One technique is to coat the heated metal with finely powdered PVC which softens under heat to form a regular surface coating. Many refrigerator and deep freeze wire shelves and trays are coated in this way.

5 **Undersealing.**
The use of bitumen (thick tar) as a coating has been used for many years to underseal cars to prevent rusting. Bitumen-impregnated tape is used around underground pipes for similar purposes.

■ A Summary of Some of the Advantages and Disadvantages of Metals

Material	Advantages	Disadvantages
Steel	High strength and stiffness. High melting point (1535°C). Easy to join. Moderately ductile (bcc).	Very poor resistance to corrosion.
Copper	Good thermal and electrical conductivity. Ductile (fcc). Easily joined. Reasonable corrosion resistance.	Expensive. Low strength. Low hardness. Work hardens extensively.
Aluminium	High strength to weight ratio. Good electrical and thermal conductivity for its weight. Ductile (fcc). Can be die-cast in alloy form. Moderate cost.	Fairly low melting point (660°C). Work hardens extensively. Difficult to join by welding or soldering without specialised fluxes or equipment.
Magnesium (normally alloyed)	High strength to weight ratio. High stiffness to weight ratio. Machines well. Can be die-cast in alloy form.	Fairly low melting point (659°C). Poor corrosion resistance. Difficult to cold form (cph). Fire risk if overheated.
Zinc (normally alloyed)	Alloys have good die-casting properties. Useful cathodic protection properties such as galvanising – its main use.	Poor strength to weight ratio. Difficult to work (cph). Expensive.

(Table continued overleaf.)

59

| Titanium | Excellent corrosion resistance. High strength to weight ratio. High melting point (1660°C). Extremely hard. | Very expensive. Very difficult to shape (cph). Specialised techniques are necessary for welding and casting. |
| Nickel | Alloyed with other metals for heat resistant properties (nimonic and nichrome). Alloyed with copper for corrosion resistant 'Monel' metal. | Too expensive for direct use. |

Fig. 5.20   The melting point of metals

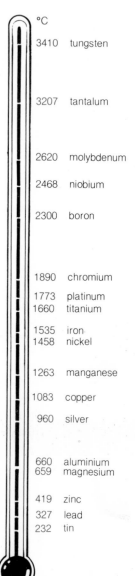

°C

3410	tungsten
3207	tantalum
2620	molybdenum
2468	niobium
2300	boron
1890	chromium
1773	platinum
1660	titanium
1535	iron
1458	nickel
1263	manganese
1083	copper
960	silver
660	aluminium
659	magnesium
419	zinc
327	lead
232	tin

6 Polymers

■ Introduction

Materials have been classified here in two simple groups; metals and non-metals. As a group, metals are distinctly different from non-metals. In the same way, non-metals have significantly similar properties which allow them to be classified together. A large proportion of non-metals which are useful to the technologist are called polymer materials. Within this grouping, the widest range of polymers is taken up by what one normally calls 'plastics', but it also includes many other equally important materials such as rubber, glass and wood.

Plasticity describes the property of a material which, when subjected to external deformation forces, enables it to remain permanently deformed after the action of the external force has been removed. In recent times a wide variety of materials have been developed which become plastic when heated. They are easily shaped into useful articles and are said to be **thermoplastic**. We must be clear about the use of the words plastic and plasticity when applied to materials. It is essential to define the property rather than use it as the name of a particular material which displays the property. Such thermoplastic materials are correctly referred to as polymers.

■ What is a Polymer?

Many words in the English language use the prefix *poly*: polygon, polyandry, polygamy. This prefix means many. *Mer* is the Greek for unit. Polymer then means many units and polymers contain from 200 units to 2000 units in the molecule. Polymer materials are chemical compounds joined together to make 'giant' or 'long chain' molecules. The main source of the raw materials is crude oil which contains various hydrocarbons. The list shows some typical hydrocarbons found in crude oil. All have different combinations of hydrogen joined to carbon.

Methane	CH_4
Ethane	C_2H_4
Propane	C_3H_8
Butane	C_4H_{10}

From such chemicals, smaller molecules are produced and can be made to react and recombine in a process called **polymerisation**. Because the resulting molecules from such a reaction are very long, they frequently become intertwined.

If you were to take a range of small samples of polymer materials and heat them carefully, below the temperature at which they start to burn, you would find that you could divide them into three distinct classes.

(a) Those that go soft and appear to melt.
(b) Those to which heat has little or no effect.
(c) Those that soften but are reluctant to melt.

(Do not attempt to try this experiment unless under the guidance of a teacher. Polymers can give off fumes which are very toxic.)

The first group are called **thermoplastics**, i.e. they soften with heat. The polymer chains may be compared to cooked spaghetti. The chains are entangled but very flexible. Polyethene, polypropylene and polystyrene are examples of thermoplastics.

The second class are called **thermosets**, i.e. they set with heat and thereafter have little plasticity. During polymerisation the molecules link side to side as well as end to end. This process called 'cross-linking' makes the material more rigid; like wire netting, the process of tying across the rows changes flexible wire into a rigid net. Polyester resin and urea formaldehyde (Formica) are thermosets.

The third group are called **elastomers** and tend to soften only slightly when heated. A limited number of cross-links allows considerable movement between chains. Rubber is an elastomer and the cross-linking can be thought of as springs, which helps to explain its elasticity.

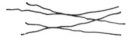 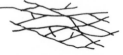 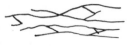

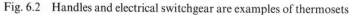

Fig. 6.1   (a) Thermoplastics   (b) Thermosets   (c) Elastomers

Fig. 6.2   Handles and electrical switchgear are examples of thermosets

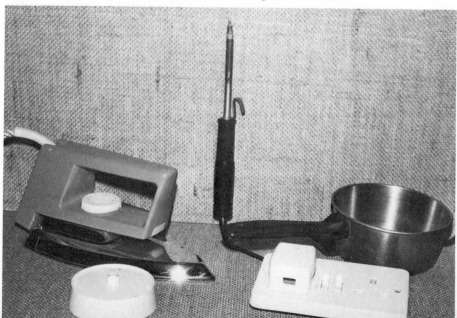

Thermoplasticity allows designers to mould materials easily and re-use offcuts and waste, which leads to economic use of materials. Thermoplastic articles are less useful where heat is involved as they lose their rigidity. Many thermoplastics soften below 100°C but there are exceptions such as PTFE which can be used up to 290°C.

For higher temperatures, thermosets are good thermal insulators and withstand heat without losing their rigidity.

■ Applications of Some Common Polymers

Chemical Name	Common Name	Uses
Poly(amide)	Nylon	Gears, bushes, bearings, curtain-rail fittings.
Poly(ethylene)	Polythene	Bottles, pipes, packaging film and bags.
Poly(propene)	Polypropylene	Chair-shells, pipes, crates.
Poly(chloroethene)	PVC	Guttering, gramophone records, cable insulation, floor covering, 'leather cloth', shoes, clothes.
Poly(methyl-2-methyl propenoate)	Polymethyl-methacrylate, Acrylic	Fluorescent light shades, signs, baths, bathroom fittings.
Poly(tetrafluoroethene)	PTFE	Non-stick coatings, low friction bearings, tape for sealing metal pipework.
Poly(phenylethene)	Polystyrene	Model kits, flower pots, disposable cups, expanded polystyrene for packaging and insulation.
Propenonitrile/buta-1, 3 diene/phenylethene co-polymer	Acrylonitrile/ butadiene/ styrene co-polymer – ABS	Refrigerator liners, cases for electrical machines, e.g. portable drills, mixers, hoovers.
Phenol methanal	Phenol formaldehyde	Iron and saucepan handles, electric plugs, lampholders.

Chemical Name	Common Name	Uses
Urea methanal	Urea formaldehyde	Electrical fittings.
Melamine methanol	Melamine formaldehyde, 'Melamine'	Decorative laminates, cups, plates.
Unsaturated polyester resin	Polyester resin	Used with glass-fibre reinforcement for boat hulls, car bodies and furniture.

Note   The first eight in this list are thermoplastics, the last four thermosets.

■ Changing the Properties of Polymers

It is common to see polyethylene sheeting that has gone hard, brittle and opaque because ultraviolet light has altered the molecular structure. To slow down this process, stabilising chemicals are added during the manufacture of the polyethylene. Disposable refuse sacks are often black in colour because carbon black additive has been added for this purpose.

Several useful changes to the properties of a polymer can be made. It can be dyed by adding pigments. It can also be 'plasticised' by adding oils or other chemicals which keep the molecular chains apart and allow them to slide more easily.

Extenders or **fillers** are additives such as chalk and wood flour which control the mechanical properties of the material and reduce material costs. The higher the proportion of filler, the greater, in general, is the strength of the article. Heat resistance is improved with the addition of mica.

Blowing agents can also be added so that, as the polymer is heated, nitrogen or carbon dioxide gas is released and a foamed polymer is produced. Expanded polystyrene for packaging, foamed polyurethane for buoyancy and polyether foams for sponges and cushioning are examples.

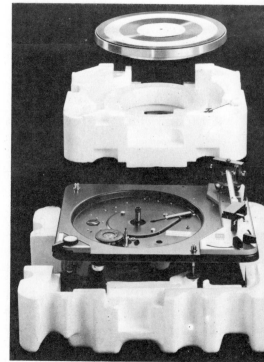

Fig. 6.3   Expanded polystyrene packaging

64

☐ Crystallinity and Amorphism

The 'spaghetti' description of polymers suggested long interwoven and jumbled chains and this random arrangement, or lack of order, is known as **amorphism**. Polymers are, however, not always amorphous but can become regularly arranged, producing **crystallinity**.

Crystallinity can be produced artificially in polymers by forcing the molecular chains to line up with each other to give an ordered molecular structure (Fig. 6.4). Crystallinity improves the directional strength and toughness of the material along the molecular chains.

In a similar way to that in which a silkworm spins a cocoon, by producing a liquid through tiny pores in its body, a spinnaret in the textile industry manufactures fibres. The fibres emerging from the fine holes of the spinnaret (Fig. 6.5) are stretched to align the molecules and so induce crystallinity.

The flexibility that can be achieved through crystallinity in polymers has led to their increasing use as simple hinges. Polymer articles with specially designed integral hinges have uses such as photographic slide boxes, disposable forceps for surgical use, and draught-strips on doors. The article is produced, often by injection moulding, to provide a uniformly rigid but amorphous structure. In the case of the draught-strip, the seam between the two parts is drawn between two dies to align the molecules in a parallel formation so as to

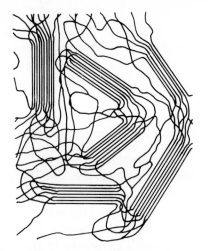

Fig. 6.4   Aligned regions of crystallinity

Fig. 6.5   Fibres emerging from a perforated plate called a 'spinnaret'

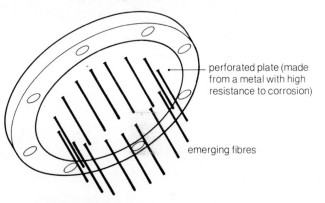

perforated plate (made from a metal with high resistance to corrosion)

emerging fibres

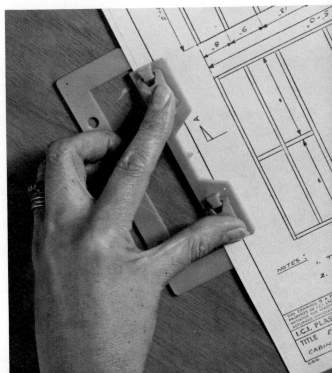

Fig. 6.6   A hole punch incorporating integral hinges

crystallise the polymer. Injection moulded integral hinges (e.g. photographic slide boxes) are commonly made by inducing the orientation of the molecules across the hinge by careful design of the mould.

■ The Temperature/Elastic Behaviour of Polymers

The thermoplastic polymers, being particularly vulnerable to moderate heat, lose their stiffness very quickly. In use, thermoplastic polymers have to be used below the temperature range that deforms them, but the deformation of polymers is important in the forming processes and allows the manufacturer to produce complex shapes.

Figure 6.7 shows the changes which take place in a thermoplastic polymer when subjected to heat. Young's modulus of elasticity is a measure of the strength of a material; when the modulus is high the material is very stiff.

Fig. 6.7   The effect of heat on a thermoplastic polymer

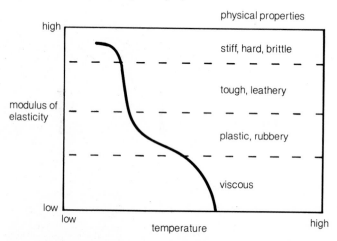

At low temperatures the polymer has properties like window glass, i.e. it is hard, brittle and very stiff. As the temperature rises, rigidity is reduced and the polymer becomes more flexible and tough. At an even higher temperature the material becomes plastic before finally turning **viscous**. A viscous material behaves like a liquid but will not pour like water; it has to be squeezed or forced to make it flow. Thick treacle is a good example of a viscous liquid. No values have been given to the modulus of elasticity or temperature range because the values vary with each individual polymer. The graph however shows the general performance of a polymer when subjected to heat.

□ Amorphous, Crystalline and Cross-linked Polymers

Figure 6.8 shows three different forms of polystyrene and how each of them is dependent upon temperature. You will recognise the performance of the

66

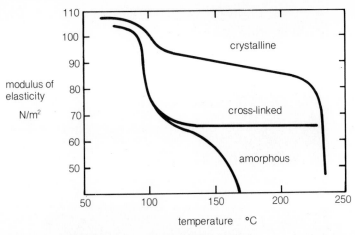

Fig. 6.8   Temperature versus elastic modulus for polystyrene

amorphous state. However, when polystyrene is in its crystalline form it stays rigid through a much greater temperature range. Suddenly it reaches its viscous stage at 235°C without passing through a long plastic stage. Because of this behaviour some of the forming processes can be made more difficult since the abrupt change in elasticity makes temperature control during forming very critical. As you would expect, the graph shows that cross-linked polystyrene loses only a little of its stiffness and then is unaffected by temperature until the level is high enough to destroy it. Elastomers behave similarly to cross-linked polystyrene but with a different temperature scale.

■ The Forming Processes

Polymers are initially produced as powders or granules. In order to shape them into finished articles they have to be heated until they become viscous and their modulus of elasticity is reduced.

■ Compression Moulding

Phenolic, urea and melamine powders are compression moulded to produce such articles as electrical switchgear, handles, etc. Thermosetting polymers are often shaped by this process.

Fig. 6.9   Compression moulding

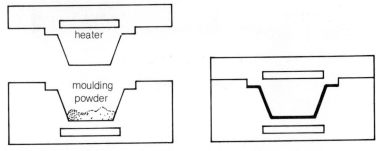

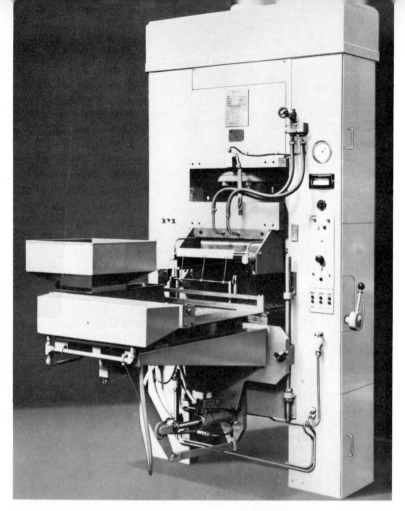

Fig. 6.10   A fully automatic compression moulding press

Fig. 6.11   Compression moulded electrical parts for domestic switches

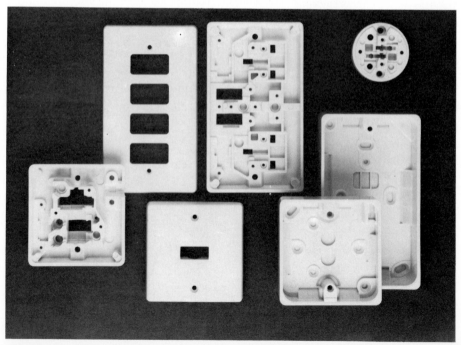

The machine consists of a hydraulic press which is used to create high pressure (approximately $7 \times 10^6\,\text{N/m}^2$) in a heated mould. The moulding powder becomes viscous under both heat and pressure and flows into the crevices of the mould while hot. Cross-links form between the polymer chains and the material 'cures' or sets hard.

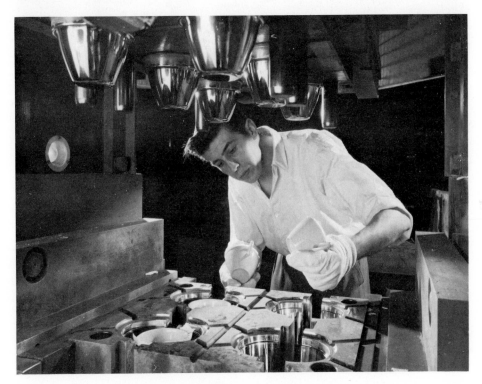

Fig. 6.12   Melamine cups being removed from a compression mould

The processing time required is substantial since the high pressure and temperature have to be maintained whilst the cross-linking reaction takes place. The articles can, on the other hand, be withdrawn from the mould whilst still hot, since the cured polymer is very rigid.

■ Injection Moulding

This process is used to mould thermoset and thermoplastic polymers. The polymer, in granule form, is heated until viscous and forced into a closed mould. Because of the viscous nature of the material, very high pressures are needed to make the polymer flow. An injection moulding machine requires pressures of approximately $7 \times 10^7\,\text{N/m}^2$, which means that the machine and locking device on the mould have to be very robust to withstand the forces involved.

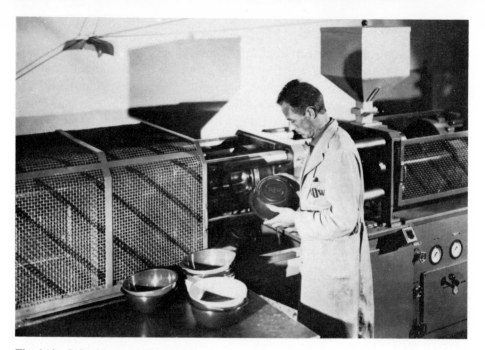

Fig. 6.13   Injection moulding polyethylene bowls

Injection moulding is suitable for a wide range of products and thermoplastic materials. The process is about six times faster than compression moulding and these fast cycle times and accuracy of moulding make it suitable for large scale production runs. Nylon combs, typewriter keys and model aircraft kits are among the articles produced by injection moulding.

Fig. 6.14   Injection mouldings in nylon

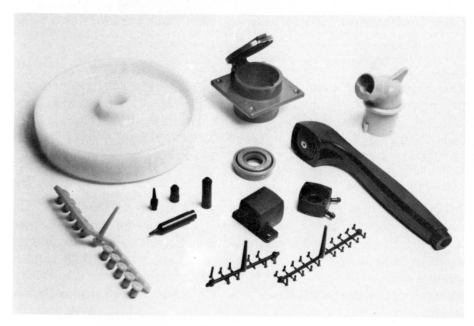

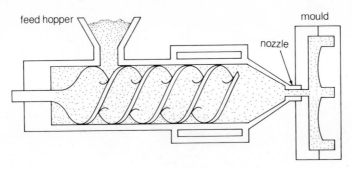

Fig. 6.15 Injection moulding

A modern injection moulding machine uses a screw to force the granules along a heated barrel. When the granules become viscous the screw is used as a plunger to force the polymer into the mould.

The moulds are generally very expensive and have to be made from high grade steel. The mould is usually highly polished to reduce friction in the flow of the viscous polymer and leave a mirror finish on the final articles. Textured moulds are used if demanded by the product design (e.g. polypropylene chairs are often textured).

■ Extrusion

Squeezing toothpaste out of a tube, or icing a cake by squeezing the icing through a forcing bag, is very similar to the extrusion process. If star shapes are to be used to decorate the cake then a star-shaped nozzle is fitted to the icing bag. In a similar way, the extrusion nozzle can be exchanged to manufacture different products.

Extrusion is one of the most widely used production processes. Thermoplastic granules are forced through a heated barrel until the viscous polymer is squeezed through the die. The product is cooled by water or air as it leaves the die and is subsequently cut to the required length.

Fig. 6.16 Extrusion

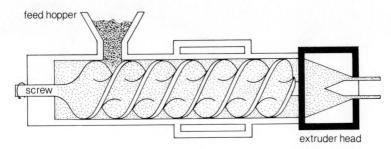

The shape of the die can be varied from a simple hole with a centrally supported core to produce tubes such as hosepipes, to very complex sections for curtain

71

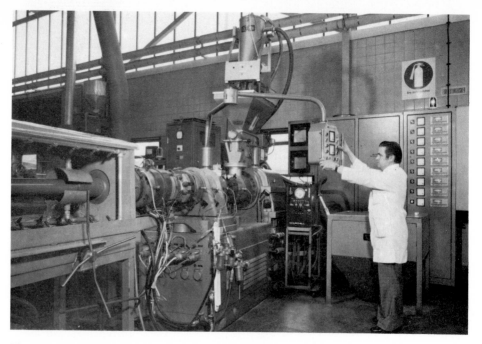

Fig. 6.17   Rigid PVC pipe being extruded and cooled by water

tracks, hollow window and door frames, and insulation for electrical copper wire. The big advantage of the process is that it produces continuous lengths as required in each production run.

Extrusion of flat sheet is another common application where continuous lengths are required. Viscous thermoplastic is extruded on to heated rotating 'calender' rolls which squeeze the material (much like a mangle does) into a continuous sheet or film. The film is cooled by air jets or a water bath before being cut to suitable lengths or reeled up.

Fig. 6.18   Calendering

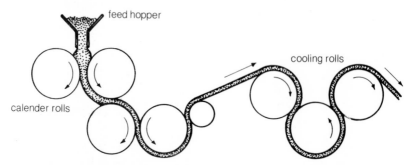

Sheet material such as coated fabrics, floor tiles, packaging laminates, decorative sheet and vinyl coated wallpapers are processed by calendering. If a textured surface is needed, as with similated leather PVC cloth, embossed rollers are used to impress their pattern on the polymer surface immediately before the sheet is cooled.

72

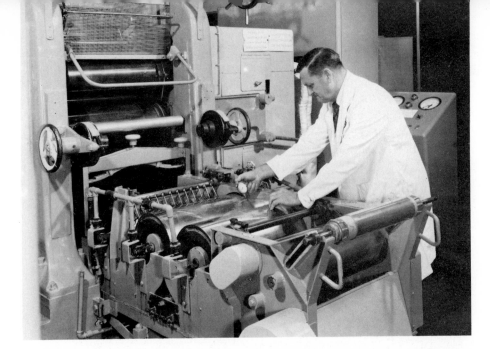

Fig. 6.19   Checking the tolerance of PVC calendered sheet

Thin film is produced by extruding a long tube and then blowing air into it continuously (while still hot) to stretch the polymer, much like blowing up a sausage-shaped balloon. After cooling, the blown tube is used to make plastic bags or split to produce flat film.

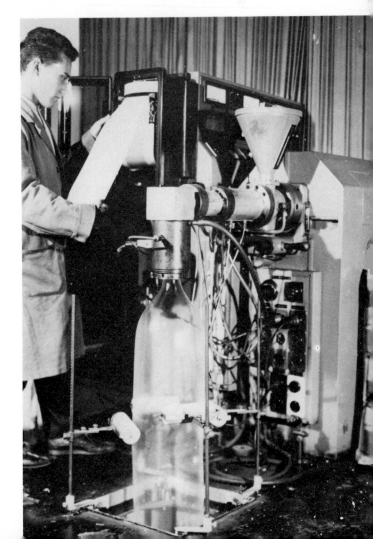

Fig. 6.20   Laboratory-scale manufacture of blown film

■ Vacuum Forming

In its simplest form, the equipment consists of a vacuum box and clamping frame, a heater and a mould. The mould, which is hollow underneath, is placed over the air outlet. Thermoplastic sheet is clamped over the mould and heated until plastic, whereupon the air is withdrawn with a vacuum pump. External air pressure pushes the thermoplastic sheet over the mould to form an accurate copy. Egg boxes, box liners, and refrigerator liners are examples of products produced by this process.

Fig. 6.21   Vacuum forming

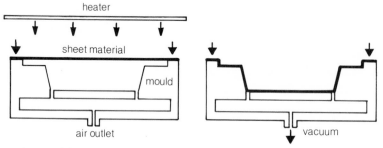

Owing to the very low pressures involved, tooling costs are low because moulds can be cheaply made from wood or plaster of Paris. However, the process is expensive because of the handling time necessary to extrude, cut, store and then reheat the sheet material. Nowadays, vacuum forming is sometimes carried out in line with a calender, so that reheating of the sheet is eliminated.

There are several disadvantages with simple vacuum-forming techniques. Firstly, the material thins out unevenly and articles tend to be wafer thin if the mould is particularly deep. This is overcome by first blowing the sheet to stretch it, and then evacuating the mould.

Fig. 6.22   A vacuum formed shower tray shell

Fig. 6.23   Blowing a sheet before evacuating the mould

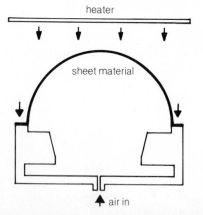

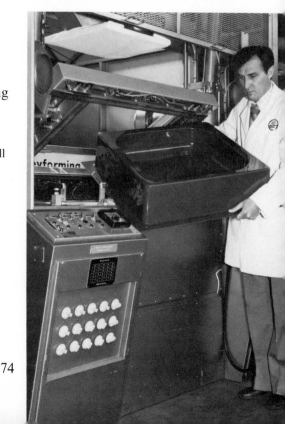

74

Secondly, the sheet is difficult to heat evenly, particularly if it is thick, since the material is such a poor conductor of heat.

Thirdly, forming is difficult with highly crystalline materials because of their sudden change to the viscous state, which means that close control of temperature is critical. Materials such as polypropylene which are highly crystalline can now be formed by a new process. The sheet is pressed in the centre by a heated die, dispensing with an overhead heater. By this method, critical temperature control can be achieved.

■ Blow Moulding

When a hollow article with a narrow neck is required, blow moulding is the technique used. Bleach bottles, squeezy bottles, large containers for storing washing-up liquid or orange juice are familiar articles produced by this method. The viscous thermoplastic is extruded into a tubular shape and is received into an open die. The die closes to seal the free end of the tube and air blows the plastic material into the moulded shape.

Fig. 6.24   Blow moulding

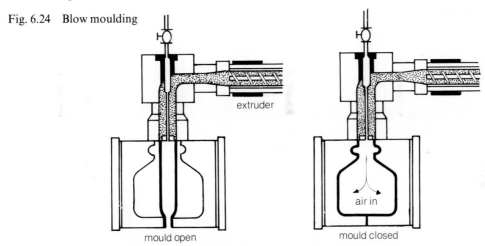

Fig. 6.25   Blow moulding PVC bottles for domestic cooking oils

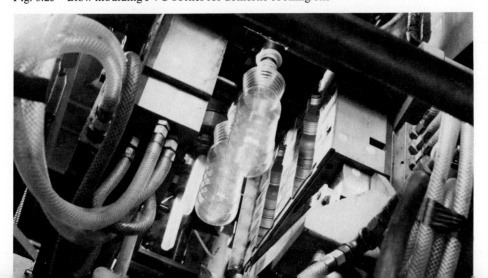

☐ The Economics of the Forming Processes

It has been mentioned that the vacuum forming of highly crystalline materials poses problems of temperature control which can make the process uneconomic for commercial operations. Other materials such as PTFE are too viscous for injection moulding and many articles are often made by a powder sintering (baking) process.

There are some processes which are more suitable for thermosets and others more suitable for thermoplastics. Occasions do arise, although rarely, where these processes are interchanged. Gramophone records are made in a copolymer containing PVC (a thermoplastic) by compression moulding, which gives improved groove definition.

Articles such as yoghurt-type tubs could be produced by injection moulding or vacuum forming. The poor flow characteristics of viscous polymers mean that injection moulding would be best to produce thick-walled tubs. Vacuum forming always stretches thermoplastic sheet and gives much thinner-walled containers. The manufacturer has to decide between thinner containers, and hence less material cost, or higher production rates.

The following table gives some of the factors which ought to be considered when comparing different processes.

	Compression moulding	Injection moulding	Vacuum forming	Blow moulding
Cost of machinery	High.	Very high.	Low.	Medium.
Cost of moulds	High.	Very high.	Low.	Medium.
Processing time	Slow.	Very fast.	Slow.	Fast.
Finishing needed	Flashing must be trimmed.	Remove the sprues, gates and runners.	Trim edges.	Trim flashing where tube has been sealed.
Difficulties with process	Possible flashing (excess material to be trimmed off).	Joint lines show where the mould splits.	Uneven thinning of sheet.	Wall thickness may vary.

It is more difficult to include extrusion in any comparison because it is a continuous process whereas the others are intermittent. Extrusion therefore has the advantages that it is more economical in terms of machine use and can produce products of intricate cross section, although it lacks the complexity of moulding that is possible with other production methods. Extrusion is used for

76

articles which are supplied in long lengths, and which will eventually be cut to size as required.

Moulding articles such as boat hulls, car bodies, etc., from glass reinforced polyester resin, is very cheap in terms of investment in machinery. However, the process is labour intensive (has to be done by hand) and is only suited to the manufacture of small quantities.

7 Rubber, Wood and Composite Materials

■ Rubber

Latex, which is processed to give natural rubber, starts as a white milky fluid produced by special cells in a variety of plants. The broken stems of some common weeds will secrete this white liquid.

'Hevea brasiliensis' is a native tree of the rain forests of the Amazon Basin in Brazil. It is cropped for latex by carefully cutting through the bark to bleed it (Fig. 7.1). Nowadays more natural rubber is produced in South East Asia (Malaysia, Indonesia) than in Brazil.

Fig. 7.1   Latex being tapped from a tree

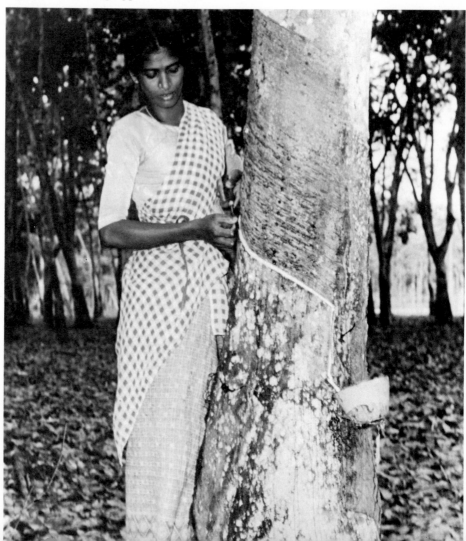

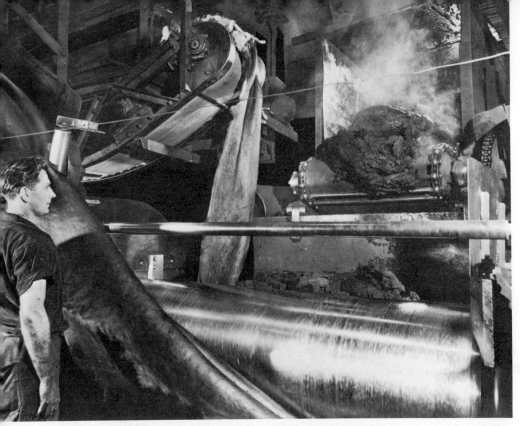

Fig. 7.2   Freshly compounded rubber being discharged onto a roll mill

In the eighteenth century, the name 'rubber' was given to the material because its chief use was to rub out pencil marks. At this time the latex could be used only as coagulated lumps rather like pieces of leather. In 1820, however, Thomas Hancock devised an apparatus which used a spiked wooden roller to work the rubber into a plastic mouldable mass. This technique is called **mastication**. In 1823 Charles Macintosh used rubber dissolved in naptha to waterproof cloth from which the 'mackintosh' raincoat was produced.

Unfortunately, progress was held back by the fact that the rubber became hard when cold and excessively sticky when warm. These are just the properties that we have come to expect of thermoplastics. It is also unfortunate that the early rubber materials perished very easily and the products developed a bad reputation.

A big breakthrough came in 1839 when Charles Goodyear discovered that by heating rubber with sulphur, the material became resistant to normal temperatures and far more durable. This process is called **vulcanisation** and is still used today.

What Goodyear was doing was making an elastomer by forming cross-links between the polymer chain. The latex molecule is a hydrocarbon (C_5H_8) known as isoprene. By introducing sulphur and heating, reactions take place to allow the sulphur to form cross-links. A large degree of cross-linking creates high rigidity in the rubber. Ebonite, for example, is a hard, brittle rubber where 25% to 40% sulphur has been added. However, vulcanisation is normally restricted to 3% by weight of sulphur and is carried out by heating the products in an atmosphere of steam or dry heat. In the tyre industry the rubber is fixed in moulds under high pressure and the mould is then heated.

Fig. 7.3   Rubber tyres and the moulds used to produce them

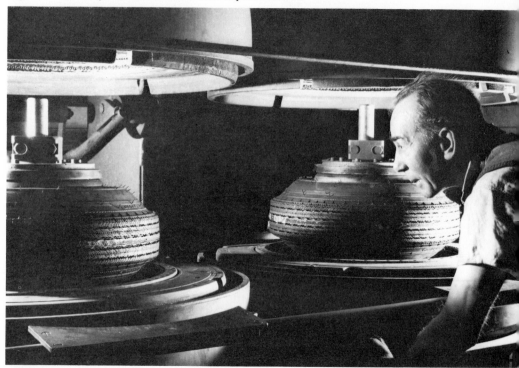

Rubber differs from any other material in its ability to regain its original shape after stretching. Rubber will often stretch up to thirteen times its original length. It can be said to have a low modulus of elasticity but a very wide elastic range. It has some plasticity as you will find if you blow up a balloon; it will not quite return to its original shape if it is taken beyond its elastic limit.

■ Synthetic Rubbers

Because of the difficulties in transporting natural rubber from Malaya during the second world war and the heavy demand for tyres for war machinery, etc., synthetic rubbers had to be developed to keep pace with demand. Since then, synthetic rubbers have been improved and their use extended to meet the requirements of advanced technology.

   Polychlorophrene, often known under the trade name of 'Neoprene' is a common synthetic rubber and is often foamed to produce a sponge-type rubber. Because of the presence of chlorine atoms in its structure, it is very resistant to solvents and has flame resistant properties.

Butyl rubber is another synthetic hydrocarbon rubber. It is widely used for inner tubes or the linings of tubeless tyres. It has the special property of being resistant to gas permeation (air leakage in these applications).

Silicone rubber is unique among the rubbers in that it contains no carbon atoms in its central chain. Instead its molecule is built around silicon and oxygen atoms. Although its mechanical properties are inferior to natural rubber at normal temperatures, at higher temperatures up to 300°C, it retains its resilience long after natural rubber has deteriorated. It is also very resistant to chemical attack and has specialised applications such as refrigeration gaskets and the fuel tank lining for Concorde.

Fig. 7.4   Shaping rubber articles   (a) Extrusion

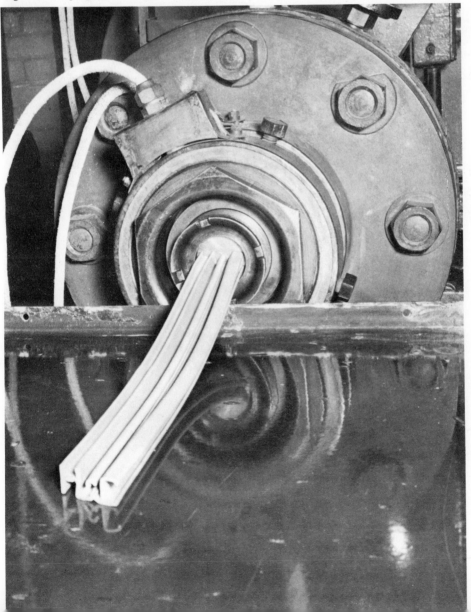

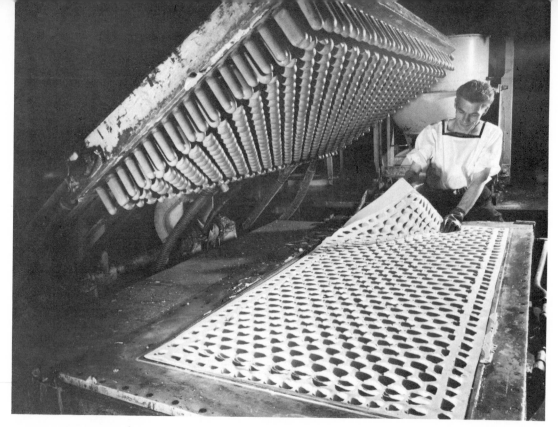

Fig. 7.4   (b) Moulding

Fig. 7.4   (c) Dipping

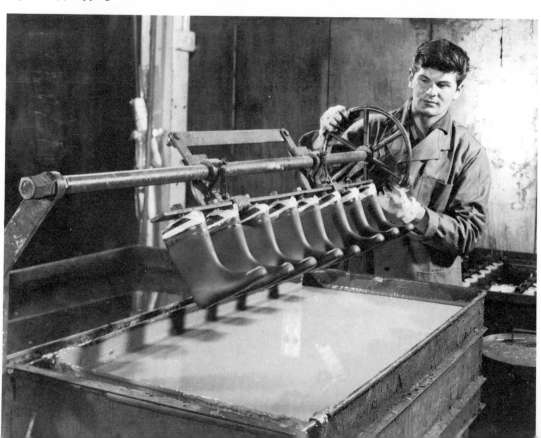

◼ Wood

The many different species of trees provide a wealth of materials which can be put to a variety of uses. Figure 7.5 gives some examples of these. Moreover, as trees can be replaced, they can be considered as a renewable source of energy.

Any material which is a natural product is inevitably variable in quality and wood is no exception. The soil and climatic conditions affect the growth rate of a tree and determine its structure, shape and strength. The ease with which wood may be cut and shaped is one of its advantages, however, the irregularity of grain, knots, warping and twisting are all disadvantages which call for some skill in shaping it. It is also vulnerable to biological attack from fungi which can cause wet rot or dry rot, whilst beetle infestation, or woodworm as it is commonly known, can also lead to serious weakening.

The trunk of a tree grows by converting glucose into cellulose. The cellulose wraps itself into a tubular cell. During the wet season, thin-walled cells with large openings are formed, these being known as the 'spring growth'. In the dry season less water is available and the cells are smaller. This 'summer growth' provides the main structural strength of the growing tree. During each growing season the tree increases its girth by both spring and summer growth and forms an 'annual ring'.

If you examine the end grain of a softwood you will see the tubular cells of the cellulose fibres. These cells are glued together with a resin called lignin which acts as a stiffening agent and protects the fibres from damage.

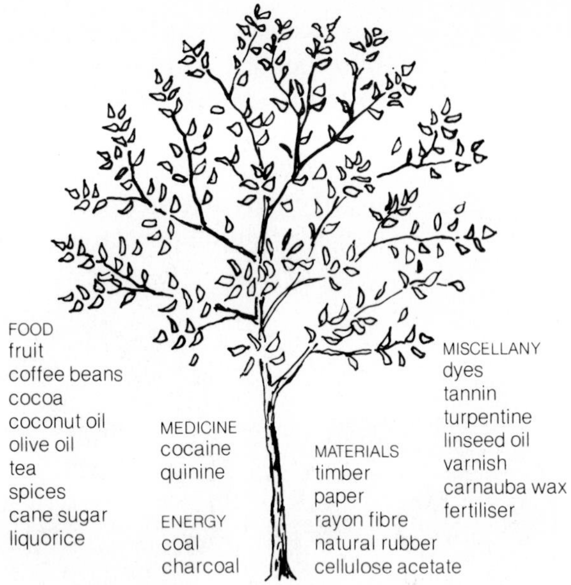

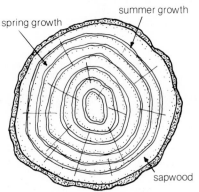

FOOD
fruit
coffee beans
cocoa
coconut oil
olive oil
tea
spices
cane sugar
liquorice

MEDICINE
cocaine
quinine

ENERGY
coal
charcoal

MATERIALS
timber
paper
rayon fibre
natural rubber
cellulose acetate

MISCELLANY
dyes
tannin
turpentine
linseed oil
varnish
carnauba wax
fertiliser

Fig. 7.5   Materials from trees

spring growth
summer growth
sapwood

Fig. 7.6   The growth of a tree
Fig. 7.7   The structure of wood

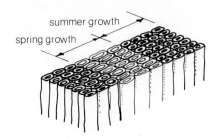

summer growth
spring growth

A material which combines two such different components, in this case a fibre bonded with resin, is known as a **composite material**. A spruce, for instance, consists of 50% cellulose, 30% lignin, 15% carbohydrates and 5% salts, waxes and resins.

The cellular structure can be modelled by lightly gluing some drinking straws together. By loading in a simple testing frame, it can be seen that such a structure can support large compressive loads.

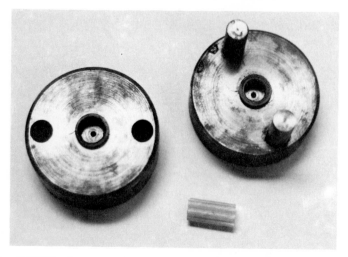

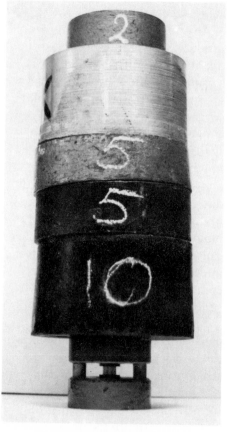

Fig. 7.8   (a) A simple compression
testing frame

(b)   Supporting a load of 33 kg

If, however, the straws were loaded across rather than along the length, the results would be dramatically weaker. When timber is used structurally, it should ideally take the load along the grain.

The amount of moisture absorbed by timber affects its properties, and reducing the moisture content increases its strength. A considerable amount of free water filling the cell cavities is removed by evaporation after the tree is felled. The remaining 25–30% of its dry weight is held within the cell walls and this has to be reduced to approximately 10% or 12% for normal uses. Evaporation by natural means, called **seasoning**, is a slow process and timber is normally seasoned in a **kiln** (oven) to speed up this process.

As timber gains moisture it expands, and when it loses moisture it contracts.

As the moisture content in the air varies with the seasons, timber will continually expand or contract.

Another problem is that the shrinking of timber leads to warping. In order to overcome these large movements, solid wood is rarely used in large panels without some provision for expansion and contraction.

Various man-made boards which minimise the effects of changing moisture content are available. **Blockboard** is constructed with strips of wood glued together with the curvature of the growth rings alternated to minimise warping. **Plywood** has alternate layers bonded together with the grain running at 90° to the adjacent layers.

Fig. 7.9   (a) Warping   (b) Blockboard   (c) Plywood

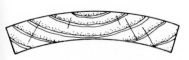
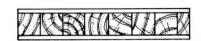
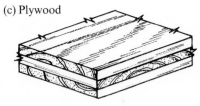

Chipboard consists of compressed particles, often graded from the coarsest in the centre of the board to almost dust particles on the outer layer. **Veneer** can then be bonded to the finely finished outer layers to give a very smooth surface finish. The adhesives used in chipboard, plywood and blockboard assist in the prevention of warping.

☐ Calculating Moisture Content

The degree of expansion of wood with increasing moisture content can be determined experimentally by measuring the size of a sample when dry and again later when it has been allowed to soak in water. The following results of a moisture content experiment were achieved by this method.

	Length (mm)	Width (mm)	Thickness (mm)	Weight (g)
Mahogany (dry)	109.1	105.5	8.1	35.9
Mahogany (wet)	109.6	108.5	8.3	45.9
Increase	0.5	3.0	0.2	10.0

The percentage increases through moisture absorption are calculated using the following formula:

$$\text{Percentage increase in length} = \frac{\text{increase in length}}{\text{length when dry}} \times 100.$$

In the above experiment the following percentage increases were calculated: length 0.46%; width 2.84%; thickness 2.46%; weight (moisture content) 27.8%.

85

Example

Figure 7.10 shows a section through an exterior panelled door made of redwood. The seasonal variations in moisture content of redwood are given in the graph.

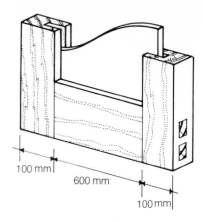

Fig. 7.10   A section through an exterior door

Fig. 7.11   The maximum and minimum moisture content of redwood

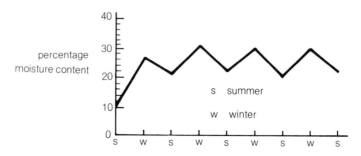

Assuming a moisture content of 10% initially, calculate the maximum change in door width to be allowed for when designing a frame to fit, taking into account variations in moisture content. For each 1% increase in moisture content, the following percentage expansions of redwood are to be used:

along the grain   0.036%;
across the grain   0.15%.

The maximum change in moisture content is 20%. Therefore the actual percentage increases are:

along the grain $0.036 \times 20 = 0.72\%$
across the grain $0.15 \times 20 = 3\%$.

Since percentage increase $= \dfrac{\text{increase in length}}{\text{length when dry}} \times 100$

the increase in length $= \dfrac{\text{percentage increase} \times \text{length when dry}}{100}$

Along the grain increase $= \dfrac{0.72 \times 600}{100} = 4.32\,\text{mm}.$

Across the grain increase $= \dfrac{3 \times 200}{100} = 6.0\,\text{mm}.$

Total increase $= 10.32\,\text{mm}.$

■ Composite Materials

When two or more materials are combined by bonding them together, they are known as **composites**. The reason for combining them is the same as for alloying metals in that it improves their mechanical or other properties. Many composites consist of reinforcing material which provides strength, bonded together in a **matrix** or glue. Wood, as you have seen, is an example of this with the strength being provided by cellulose fibres, bonded in a matrix of lignin.

■ Layer Composites

Layer composites, or **laminates** as they are more commonly known, are widely used to improve the toughness of materials. Formica and melamine are common layer composites of paper and melamine formaldehyde resin. The resin itself, like most thermosets, is very brittle and is toughened with alternate layers of paper which consist of cellulose fibres. The uppermost layer of paper is often coloured or patterned and is then covered with a final coat of clear resin which provides the hard heatproof surface. The whole sandwich is heated in a press for the resin to cure and form cross-links.

   Rayon fibre (a reconstituted cellulose fibre from wood pulp) is widely used in the textile industry for clothing, and also in the tyre industry, when rayon cloths form the reinforcing material for the side-wall of the modern motorcar tyre.

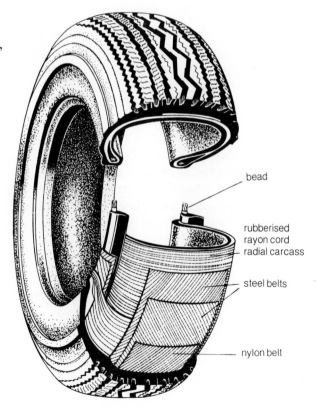

Fig. 7.12   The structure of a modern
             motorcar tyre

bead

rubberised
rayon cord
radial carcass

steel belts

nylon belt

Glass reinforced plastic (GRP) laminates are used to produce canoes, boat hulls and some car bodies. Toughness is achieved by using strands of glass fibre which are elastic. The maximum amount of glass fibre and the minimum quantity of polyester thermosetting resin produce the strongest laminate. Carbon fibre can be similarly used with polyester resin for reinforcement, though at present it is much more expensive than glass fibre.

'Tufnol' is the product name of a layer composite consisting of woven linen impregnated with phenolic resin. It has applications as gears, bearings and slides in machinery where loadings are moderately light.

Sandwich panels of a hollow polymer skin filled with a foamed plastic core combine high rigidity with low weight.

Layer composites are not restricted to polymers. Metals can also be laminated though the reasons for doing so may differ. A stainless steel saucepan with a copper base combines the thermal properties of copper with the hardness and non-corroding properties of stainless steel.

Metal laminates are also used in special applications as bimetallic strips. As the temperature of the strip increases, the greater expansion of one metal causes the strip to bend elastically. This can be used to make or break an electrical contact.

■ **Particle Composites**

As the name implies, the composite consists of combined particles. The most common particle composite is concrete which consists of coarse particles of gravel or crushed stone, fine particles of sand, and the bonding matrix of cement. These three constituents are thoroughly mixed together and water added. The cement sets by reacting with water and binds the reinforcing particles together.

Concrete has a high compressive strength but low tensile strength. When used as a beam, the upper surface is in compression while the lower surface is in tension. In order to make the beam more resistant to bending, steel rods (which are strong in tension) can be embedded in the concrete for further reinforcement. This is called **reinforced concrete**.

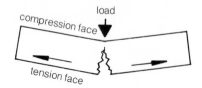

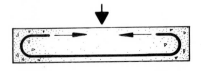

Fig. 7.13　(a) Concrete under stress

(b) Reinforced concrete— the hooked ends of the reinforcing steel transfer the load from the reinforcement to the concrete

The rubber used in car tyres is mixed with fine particles of carbon black. These particles serve to reinforce the rubber and increase its resistance to cracking and ultraviolet damage. If sufficient carbon black is added, the rubber can conduct electricity. This has uses where static electricity is a problem, e.g. the rubber trolley wheels used in operating theatres will earth this static electricity more easily.

The reflective properties of modern car number plates are achieved by cementing glass beads to an aluminium backing sheet with a clear or coloured polymer matrix.

8 Materials Selection and the Future

■ Materials Selection

The selection of a material or materials for a product is seldom easy, whether it is a simple object like a hinge or a complex machine such as a car. Making the decision is an essential part of the design process and depends very much on the skill and experience of the designer.

There are three main factors affecting the choice. All of these are interrelated.

Fig. 8.1   The three main factors influencing materials selection

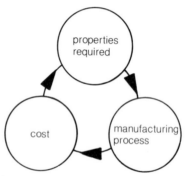

1   Properties required.
    The engineer or designer faced with a choice will ask many questions in order to understand the task that the product has to perform. Does it have to withstand heat? Will it be in a corrosive environment? Is the weight important? How strong does it have to be? The answers to such questions define the properties of materials required. The designer is then in a position to narrow his choice of materials.

2   Manufacturing process.
    There are often different ways of making a component (e.g. cast, sintered, or fabricated). The method of manufacture and the material have to be chosen together so that they are compatable. As a simple example, consider a metal window frame which may be made from steel or aluminium. While a steel section would have to be rolled to achieve the desired shape, the lower shaping forces necessary for aluminium allow extrusion as a suitable manufacturing process. The choice of material also determines the joining methods and the surface finish. A steel frame would be galvanised and then painted, whereas aluminium may be anodised.

90

3   Cost.

This is fundamental to the manufacture of any product. There is little point in making a perfect object if it costs so much that no one will buy it. It may be necessary to reduce the quality of the new material (or adopt a cheaper method of manufacture) to enable it to be made at a price which people are prepared to pay. This can be clearly seen in the case of car exhaust systems. It is perfectly possible to make a stainless steel exhaust which will last indefinitely. Most people, however, buy a mild steel system, knowing that they will have to replace it in one to two years. Why? Because it costs much less.

It should be realised that although these three factors have been discussed separately, the choice of material will usually be a compromise between them. In some cases the function (i.e. the properties) will be the most important. In many more cases the cost will be the critical factor. Thus the 'best' material for any situation can only be found when all the data has been collected and considered.

■ Looking to the Future

It is almost impossible to assess what the materials situation will be in the future, since it depends on so many unknown factors. What is certain, however, is that raw materials will never again be so readily available or so cheap as they have been in the past. There will be a definite shortage of all materials. An important factor in this is that minerals are becoming more and more difficult to extract as accessible deposits become worked out.

Fig. 8.2   The energy required to produce 1 m³ of material

energy requirements   MJ/m³

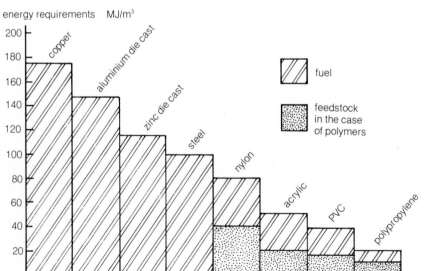

At one time it was thought that polymers might be the answer to many of our problems. The low energy consumption involved in producing them make polymers an attractive alternative to metals. However, being predominately hydrocarbons, the raw materials from which they are made are controlled by current world prices for oil. The escalation in oil prices through the 1970s forced us to reflect on the way we use oil. The industrialised world presently uses 22 million barrels of oil a day. By the year 2000 it is estimated that Europe's requirements alone could exceed this figure. It is now realised, therefore, that using oil as a raw material for polymers is limited, and although polymers are useful they by no means solve all our needs as far as material resources are concerned.

Perhaps the most definite point that may be made about the future is that modern society must curb wasteful use of materials. We have become known as the 'throw-away society'. Instead of repairing an article, it is often thrown away and replaced. The arguments for this are based on economics rather than material resources, and it is inevitable that thought will need to be given to altering this approach.